HEALING PRESENCE
THE ESSENCE OF NURSING

JoEllen Koerner, RN, PhD, FAAN, and CEO, NurseMetriX, is an author, editor, speaker, researcher, educator, and nurse executive leader who is well known for her efforts to foster high standards in nursing.

She is a former President of the American Organization of Nurse Executives and the recipient of the Lifetime Distinguished Service Award from the AONE Institute for Patient Care Research and Education. Dr. Koerner has had extensive executive level management/leadership experience in health care administration, education, regulation, and e-commerce.

She has written three books, numerous articles, and also served as Editor or Board Advisor on multiple nursing journals; *Nurse Week, Nursing Administration Quarterly, Nursing Outlook, Journal of Nursing Administration, Journal of Nursing Education, Nursing Spectrum,* and *Journal of Professional Nursing.*

Dr. Koerner has also served on many national Advisory Boards including Robert Wood Johnson, Johnson & Johnson, PEW Health Professions, National Commission on Nursing Implementation Project, Picker Institute, Fetzer Institute, HillRom Center for Nursing Leadership, Community-Campus Partnerships for Health, International Center for Nursing, American Academy of Nursing, and the American Association of Colleges of Nursing. In the United States, she has consulted at Pine Ridge Reservation. Internationally, her work has included consultations in New Zealand, Australia, and the Philippines, as well as to the Ministry of Health, Prague, Czechoslovakia. Her international and voluntary work is currently focused on web-enhanced workforce development for underrepresented sectors of society.

In addition to this edition of *Healing Presence*, Dr. Koerner has a number of related materials and resources available including:

- her book, *Mother, Heal My Self*
- Values Profile with Interpretation
  - Individual
  - Group
  - Organization/Association
- On-line In-Sight! Classes
- Healing Presence Classes
  - On-line
  - Teaching Packet
- Healing Presence Visual Homeopathy Card Collection
- Presentations and Consultations

For more information contact: jkoerner@globalnursingnetwork.org

HEALING PRESENCE
THE ESSENCE OF NURSING

JoELLEN KOERNER, RN, PhD, FAAN

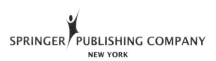

SPRINGER PUBLISHING COMPANY

NEW YORK

Watson Caring
Science Institute

Springer Publishing Company, LLC
11 West 42nd Street
New York, NY 10036
www.springerpub.com

Acquisitions Editor: Allan Graubard
Senior Production Editor: Diane Davis
Composition: S4Carlisle Publishing Services
Cover Design: David Levy
Cover Illustration: "Inner World" is a visual homeopathy image created by renowned graphics artist David Stirts. It is part of the Healing Presence Visual Homeopathy collection. David may be contacted about his art work as well as customized imagery at: http://platonicarts.com

ISBN: 978-0-8261-0754-1
E-book ISBN: 978-0-8261-0755-8

11 12 13 14 15/5 4 3 2 1

The author and the publisher of this work have made every effort to use sources believed to be reliable to provide information that is accurate and compatible with the standards generally accepted at the time of publication. Because medical science is continually advancing, our knowledge base continues to expand. Therefore, as new information becomes available, changes in procedures become necessary. We recommend that the reader always consult current research and specific institutional policies before performing any clinical procedure. The author and publisher shall not be liable for any special, consequential, or exemplary damages resulting, in whole or in part, from the readers' use of, or reliance on, the information contained in this book. The publisher has no responsibility for the persistence or accuracy of URLs for external or third-party Internet Web sites referred to in this publication and does not guarantee that any content on such Web sites is, or will remain, accurate or appropriate.

Library of Congress Cataloging-in-Publication Data
Koerner, JoEllen Goertz.
    Healing presence / JoEllen Koerner. — 2nd ed.
       p. ; cm.
    Includes bibliographical references and index.
    ISBN 978–0–8261-0754–1
    1. Nursing—Psychological aspects.   2. Healing—Psychological aspects.   3. Holistic nursing.
4. Nurse and patient.   I. Title.
    [DNLM: 1. Nursing Care—methods.   2. Mind–Body Therapies—nursing. WY 100]
    RT86.K626 2011
    610.73—dc22   2010050433

Printed in the United States of America by Bang Printing.

This book is dedicated to the Universal Spirit that unites and heals us all.

CONTENTS

SECTION IV
A HEALING FIELD: THE CONTEXT FOR NURSING PRACTICE

FOREWORD
REFLECTIONS OF A NURSE HEALER

> *... and at the end of all our exploring will be to arrive where we started ... and to know the place for the first time.*
>
> T. S. Elliot
> *Little Gidding*

All nurses, regardless of their career path, have at one time or another enjoyed the privilege of sharing our healing presence with patients. This opportunity to contribute to the patient's health and well-being using compassion and empathy has been what most nurses would say drew them into the profession. This "call" to our work, acknowledged as timeless, has not really had the center stage it might, given its magnetic pull to the profession. In fact, in my 35 years as a nurse, I have seen the topic of the essence of nursing discussed more when the profession was near a drought either in recruits or in role satisfaction. Our cyclical conversations have been inadequate for such an important cornerstone of nursing work. It seems the energy so needed to fuel the profession lies deep in this aspect of our work. How we can collectively learn to use it more effectively is the key.

DRILLING DOWN TO THE ESSENCE ...

I have often viewed and described the work of nursing in two dimensions: "doing" and "being." All nurses understand the "doing" dimension of nursing. So much of a nurse's preparation, socialization, and role definition lie in what we do. The "doing" skills and technical accountabilities are that which keep nurses running and busy. This dimension of nursing work has clearly changed, grown, and become more complex over time. "Doing" is clearly more concrete, able to be measured, and generally what has been perceived to be valued.

The "being" dimension of the role of nurse is less about what nurses do and more about the how. The focus of "being" and how the nurse comes to the bedside receives less time in a nurse's preparation, socialization, and even role definition. Admittedly, this "being" dimension is more difficult to describe, harder to measure, and although valued by nurses and those patients who benefit from it, has not always been at the center of what is rewarded. "Being" is what slows down the nurse so that space is created for an authentic, deep connection with the patient and healing. The work of "being" has remained constant over time. Embedded in the "being" dimension of the role lies the essence of nursing, and it is here that the call to the profession is actualized.

One might say, over my career, I have had a preoccupation and conversation around the essence of nursing. When years have passed since I have seen certain colleagues and we end up in conversation about nursing, I am certain they say, "she's still at it." I even bore myself at times. Nevertheless, bringing focus and language to this "being" dimension has been my lifelong work. Ten years into my nursing career while in graduate school, I fell deep in the study of the humanistic psychologists, particularly Carl Rogers. His theories and writings on *Becoming a Person* and *Person Centered Approach* brought me a new perspective on the "being" aspect of my bedside practice. The biggest shift was looking inward at myself first before looking at how I might be more effective in working with others. Rogers' delineation of the conditions necessary for this deep connection with patients gave me a loom to weave the threads of my work around "being" into. These conditions of genuineness, acceptance, and empathetic understanding were fitting for the preparation of coming to the bedside to be fully present for the patient. One might even say, as nurses, these conditions are obligatory in occupying the space for healing with patients.

As nurses, we have been taught and have learned a fair amount about the importance of empathy. We have witnessed its effect on patients, learned from our experiences, and nurses have earned well-deserved credibility in its delivery. We have spent little time, however, on individual development of genuineness and acceptance. It is as if once we've received the call into nursing it was assumed that these two later conditions were in place. Nurses, as great as we might be in the eyes of those we serve, are as human as anyone. As such, we come with our own individual work as we journey toward our potential. Seated so close to the patient in the practice of nursing, this individual obligation takes on crucial importance.

The condition of being genuine in our relationships with patients and others seems welcoming. What an invitation to be who I am, which is not as simple at times as it may seem. Besides acknowledging our humanness, being genuine implies a deep awareness and knowing of self. Moreover, it calls for an appreciation of self with all the beauty and bruises that our true self reflects. The acceptance of our self as imperfect creates the capacity to be more open, transparent, and vulnerable. This authenticity plays a key role in how we are seen and experienced by others. Being genuine is a necessary condition in order for others to be real with us.

I have found Rogers' second condition of acceptance dependent on the capacity to be genuine. When I am accepting of my true self, I am more accepting of others and where they are. Just as self-acceptance implies being free from preconceived notions about myself, accepting others requires the giving up of any bias or predetermined perceptions about where others should be. This means no prejudice, labels, or judging of others. Only when we are fully accepting of our true self, we are able to be fully open to accepting others. The gift of acceptance is the nurturant space it creates for others to discover more of their true self.

One can easily see how development of nurses' capacity for genuineness and acceptance influences their capacity for Rogers' third condition of empathetic understanding. The ability to understand and to feel the patients' journey, struggle, and emotions, as they are experiencing them, is the ultimate privilege of the role of nurses. This is not new territory for nurses. Capacity, however, will be enhanced, perhaps even transformed with a deeper self-knowledge, acceptance, and new awareness.

This journey with self opens one's eyes to see new potential. We as nurses can, and will, imagine the impact it could have in serving patients. Can we imagine at the same time the new potential and energy that would be created with renewed wholeness in nurses and nursing? The answer lies in our individual and collective willingness to claim, embrace, and become our essence, one nurse at a time.

> Walk slowly with intent, courage, and a sense of inquiry through the pages of wisdom that follow. Joellen Koerner, one of nursin's most entrusted friends and healers, is our guide to discovery and coming home.

Julie MacDonald, RN, MSN
Chief Operating Officer
St. Joseph Mercy Healthcare System

PREFACE
AN INVITATION

O ur daughter, Kristi, was 29 and in the prime of her life. Young and beautiful, moving up the corporate ladder at Citibank, happily married with a healthy and active child of her own, Kristi was living the American Dream. Suddenly, a complex pregnancy laced with a series of medical errors threatened her very existence. I quit my position as chief nursing officer of a large health system and took her and the new baby into our home. For the next 9 months, we would live a life–death drama that changed our world forever.

What would you do if your child was injured by a profession that has been the source of meaning and purpose for all of your life? How would you respond as one error led to another, until suddenly the very existence of your beloved child lay in the balance? Where would you go to help reverse the situation when the health care industry, the seemingly obvious solution, was also the problem?

Living on the Midwest Prairie for my entire life, I have a special love and appreciation for the Sioux Nation who live in South Dakota. It was their loving support and kind invitation to take part in their healing practices that restored Kristi to health, and more importantly, both of us to wholeness. (That story and the series of e-mail messages from Wanigi Waci, a Lakota spiritual healer, which depict their "science," were captured in another book entitled *Mother, Heal My Self: An Intergenerational Healing Journey Between Two Worlds*.) In that dance between both worlds, I came to understand the innate capacity for the human spirit to transcend adversity and heal not only the body/mind/spirit but also the issues and patterns that extend for generations within a family story. Most importantly, it was in that space that I learned what it means to be a healing presence in this world.

Kristi recovered over a period of 7 years. And it was during those years that I set out to "understand" what had transpired. All the models of science and healing that were such an important part of my socialization into nursing were true but partial. I studied with a medicine man and a quantum physicist from MIT, comparing their mental models on "how the world works." I read extensively in the fields of quantum science, psychology, philosophy, and metaphysics. I interviewed 200 RNs to understand what it is that makes their work difficult. When they arrive at work with the intent of providing quality care, what fosters a medical error? The understandings of this deep inquiry led to the writing of this book.

Through a long and rewarding career in nursing, I have been privileged to support and learn from many about the wellness–illness patterns that mark the human experience. It is frequently an illness event that slows us down, inviting us to step outside normal routines to reevaluate the beliefs and patterns that create the life we live. Cares of the day become insignificant when one is confronted with one's mortality. The focus shifts to the deeper questions of the soul.

Occasionally when we are "ill," we are fortunate enough to have the support and safety of a caring relationship in which we can ponder with vulnerability and reflect with candor on our fundamental beliefs, assumptions, and expectations for ourselves and others. We begin to sort through the panorama of lived experiences we have encountered and discern how we have used them to understand and ascribe meaning to life as a whole and our life specifically.

While the art and science of nursing have long been recognized as the hallmark of the health profession, it is the *presence of the nurse that is central to the discipline.* The intent and commitment that bring them to their vocation is the heart of their professional performance. When there is congruence between who they are and what they do, nurses bring their soul to work. This authenticity is experienced as a healing presence that potentiates the patient's self-healing capacity. Both the nurse and patient experience meaning in their exchange and each becomes whole.

This book is designed to place 21st century nursing into a timeless paradigm, one that transcends the economic, political, and technological culture of the day. It is important to remember that nursing is a social mandate and has been part of the communal fabric since the dawning of civilization. Birth, death, and health–illness are a part of the legacy of humankind, which requires the assistance of others. Exciting developments in science and technology have made the role of a nurse richer and more complex. We now have an array of tools and services to offer those we care for that were not available for our predecessors. However, the unifying, underlying essence of our work is the timeless and profound healing presence we offer, which enhances the exploration and creation of meaning in the inevitable health challenges faced by individuals, families, and groups whose lives we are privileged to serve.

The truth of that knowing is shared in the first section of this book through a case study of healing between two cultures: contemporary Western Allopath and Native Healing. Aspects of Kristi's healing journey are shared through a series of exemplars and e-mails written by Wanigi Waci as he explained the science behind the healing paradigm used by a Medicine Man. This offers an opportunity for you to increase your awareness of other ways of knowing/healing practiced in cultures different from, but profoundly relevant to, the mainstream culture of healing in America today. Such awareness is central to nursing in the postmodern world, expanding perception that fosters In-Sight! Wisdom generated by intuitive creativity, as much as data gathered through logical analysis, must be the guide for clinical practice in the postmodern world.

Other sections in this book are grouped into various orientations that may best fit your particular interests or worldview. The second section explores new models for transpersonal caring through the lens of philosophy, spirituality, and complexity science. It examines the bioenergetic body—the "five bodies" that comprise the amazing human being. Ways to "assess the intangible" are also considered as we expand our work to be more inclusive. The physiology and philosophy behind healing presence are also examined, along with nursing practices that potentiate its power on behalf of those we serve each day. For those wanting a "quick" understanding, the tenets of healing are offered in summary boxes. Those wanting a deeper understanding of the science behind the precept can read the more extensive dialogue that follows.

The next section of this book explores authentic presence and ways of knowing. When we live the values that are central to our lives, we experience balance in our personal situation, mastery in our professional career, and self-empowered leadership in managing our life path as an expression of our soul's destiny. From this centered space, we are open to multiple ways of knowing, seeing, and being, which foster creativity, innovation, and the simple joy of existence.

For the quintessential nurse scholar, the final section of this offering focuses on the unfolding discoveries of quantum physics and our understanding of health and illness from the new science perspective. It explores principles of art and how we intuitively apply them to the body beautiful as we assess its perfections/imperfections and the shifting patterns that guide our clinical practice. The grand "awakening" of the human race is also explored in a mini tour of the differing eras in our epic journey toward understanding what it means to be human.

The essence of "Authentic Presence" experienced by others in the service rendered by nursing requires an exchange of the human spirit; in the juncture of body–mind–spirit, a synthesis of wholeness is grasped. The underlying philosophy expressed in this book reflects an appreciation of, and a place for, all aspects of life and human endeavor. Because life is so big, and the world is becoming increasingly small, the beliefs and values of all we serve in nursing are asking to be recognized, respected, and honored in our awareness and our healing work.

Where theories come and go in just a few centuries or even decades, inklings of the mystical are found in the writings of great personalities the world over. People such as Einstein, William Blake, and Carl Jung have demonstrated that deep thought is always inspired from within. Their reflections are woven throughout the scientific exploration undertaken here as an effort to interweave the philosophical and spiritual into our predominant scientific frame of reference.

Growing up in a small rural community of 1000 people, I discovered the power of the written word. I quickly learned that, through a book, one could engage in an inner dialogue with people across time and distance. This book is not meant to be a comprehensive scientific review but, rather, an introduction to conversations with some of the finest minds in existence. It is a small effort to introduce you to my friends (as noted in the many footnotes inviting you to join their dialogue). It is an invitation to remember your call to nursing, to reengage with the passion and commitment that inspired you. It is a statement of gratitude for all you have contributed to the life of humankind, in general, and mine, in particular. It is a celebration of the power of the human spirit that is manifest everywhere we practice. And it is a statement of gratitude to All-That-Is for the privilege of sharing the life journey with so many at this time in history.

> *Ask that I may be forgiven if my pen*
> *has gone astray or my foot has slipped,*
> *for to plunge into the abyss of the Divine*
> *Mysteries is a perilous thing and no easy*
> *task is it to seek to discover the Unclouded*
> *Glory which lies behind the veil.*
>
> Al-Ghazali

ACKNOWLEDGMENTS

A debt of gratitude is expressed to all who have gone before, created the current path who have that is unfolding. I am indebted to Dr. Bruce Fisher and Donna Ehrenreich for their wisdom, insight, and candor in shaping the manuscript. Heartfelt appreciation goes to Allan Graubard for focusing and refining my voice. Deep admiration is extended to David Stirts for creating beautiful illustrations and tapestries that reflect the essence of concepts being considered. Profound respect and gratitude is held for Wanigi Waci and the Wase Wakpa community for their unconditional love and generosity in sharing their world with Kristi and I, and all of humanity. Finally, and foremost, profound appreciation and devotion are felt for my personal and professional families whose love, guidance, and unconditional support have been a sustaining and inspiring presence in my life.

A disclaimer:
Many quotes offered in this book have been collected throughout my career from presentations, writings, and conversations with colleagues and kept in a small file in my desk called "Inspiration." While I cannot always find the originating source of these encouraging messages, when possible I have provided the author's names as an invitation to the reader to explore their wise and rich words.

Section I

A Healing Story
Exploring the Lived Experience

You think we are human beings having a spiritual experience.
In our way, we see people as spiritual beings
Having a human experience.

Wanigi Waci

CHAPTER 1

NURSING
A SACRED WORK

To possess the will that nurses our visions and brings us closer to the path of angels, that infuses us with compassion and makes us glow like a soft amber—that is the secret of sacred wisdom.

Henryk Skolimowsji

The profession of nursing is a tribe, complete with its own culture, customs, and mores. Early tribal groups found strength and flexibility through the differentiation of task and orientation as hunter gatherers, artisans, and healers shared in caring for the needs of the community. So too, contemporary nursing is offered by practitioners with a bias for the rigors of science, the aesthetics of artistic expression, or the meaning of spiritual orientation. Individually and collectively, our differences converge on a shared mission: the support of healing on this planet. This book is an invitation to examine our world and our work from the multiple perspectives of our clan.

Diversity is the strength of our profession. On the vast Dakota Prairie, an interesting phenomenon is observed. The eastern part of the state is agricultural in nature with vast fields of corn, soybeans, and wheat covering the earth. In the heat of summer, rows of yellow sunflowers rotate their heads to follow the sun in days of endless succession. Divided by the Missouri River, the western side of the state comprises miles of unbroken prairie with multiple varieties of foliage blanketing the rolling hillside. Drought may wipe out an entire field of corn in a dry year, while the prairie hosts a specific type of cover. A wet year may drown that same field of corn, while the prairie hosts a completely different look as other grasses or flowers flourish in the diversity of that environs. The prairie is prepared for any occasion, while the fields with only one option often find conditions less than ideal.

One of the many joys of the profession is that our work is needed in areas of education, service, or research. We can express our skill and knowledge in tertiary care, in business, or in the community. There is even diversity in the timing of our job; nights or weekends anyone? Young professionals often move around to opportunities that expand their capacities. A mother balances children with a career, while an older nurse reduces hours to care for an aging parent. We can step in and out of the work as the demands of life dictate. But always and forever, the need for supporting the health of society remains. Our calling and the work it entails are perennial. It is a distinct privilege to be a nurse!

Healing presence is the difference between safety and quality. Innovation and creativity are central to the quality movement. A nurse who is totally present sees the subtle, perceives the whole, and co-creates with the person—and the health team—a creative response to the uniqueness of the situation. The higher good of all is served.

A RETURN OF THE FEMININE HEALING ENERGY

We are living in a most extraordinary and opportune time as the world faces a crucial juncture in the history of humankind. The last Renaissance focused on the merging of art and science—the creativity and wisdom of others. However, this current awakening includes the illumination of our own personal artistic expression and philosophy, the embracing of our own capacity and wisdom. We are poised to come home to ourselves, embracing and expressing the authentic essence of our own "wholeness."

As we continue movement into the new millennium, some of us sense that this is a major turning point in the long human journey. We are beginning to perceive the difference between the superficial and the substantive, to recognize what is being born while surrounded by what is dying. An alert mind will identify new potential as old things fall away. To witness life at this level, we must view the process from soul territory. Fortunately, we are no stranger here. This is the very center of the nursing domain.

The epoch of nursing began with the inhalation of the first breath of humankind. It is a story of presence and support, a story defined by witness and engagement, a story pregnant with compassion and caring. Ours is a story filled with ethos, intrigue, breakthroughs and setbacks, moments of beauty, and periods of darkness. It is a story of the feminine healing energy moving through the ages, a story that reveals the pattern of watchfulness, the practice of seeing and being seen by the Source.

Every being has access to both masculine and feminine energy. The feminine or yin includes such attributes as receptive, intuitive, inward, sensitive, delicate, emotional, and nurturing. The masculine or yang includes such attributes as outward, hard, firm, logical, strong, rational, rough, and loud. Although both yin and yang are essential to living a life in dynamic balance, the core of nursing practice lies within the subtle feminine healing energy of *active receptivity*—to see fully, take in, and support the whole with a compassionate, caring heart.

The ever-expanding field of health care has primarily focused on masculine qualities of medicine, which is nested within this oft unseen field of feminine energy—a most essential element in the healing journey. Bearing witness to others with a consciousness of *healing presence* creates a sacred space filled with nonjudging and nonscripted energetic expectation. It is simply "being with" the other. Our presence provides a "source of mercy that helps others untie their tangles" (Brisken, 2005). This is the ultimate, the primary but often overlooked function of nursing practice. By offering compassionate care in a deeply mindful manner, the healing potential that resides within the other is released.

This way of seeing and being requires a specific responsibility for watching over things of the soul. Such a witness plunges us into the farthest reaches of perception and consciousness. Seeing fully takes us to the essence of our higher selves, that which is our sacred connection point to All-That-Is. From this portal, we become fully aware that there is *something we all know*, which simultaneously deepens our identification with others and the very earth itself. We come alive with feeling, recognizing the unbroken field of energetic consciousness that creates a vibration of shared meaning, flowing as an expression of heart, mind, and will. This is the *essence of wholeness, our sacred oneness*.

Facilitating an open and safe environment prompts an apprehension of wholeness, which is the receptive feminine function in the universe. Reb Zalman observed (as cited in Briskin, 2005, p. 9):

> The other thing that is necessary is to have women involved. Because it's in the nature of the masculine vision to see the figure and ignore the ground. In other words that which is erect and that which enters and that which has power, and that which deposits sperm, and that which is active, and so on and so forth.

There is too often an ignoring of those who receive, or contain, or hold. Much focus is placed on the object, leaving little awareness of the field in which it sets. One sees the black letters on the page without conscious recognition of the white space that surrounds them. In health care settings, the doctor is the episodic visitor, while nursing is a 24-hour presence. And yet, it is medicine, without the inclusion of nursing, that society references when health care issues are debated publically. Zalman continues:

> I can't see the wind, but I see the flag in the wind. . . . Despite that I don't see the wind, I see the flag moving. I understand that what I'm seeing is not just the flag, but its flag and wind. . . . In similar fashion when I look at a river, it's the bed and it's the water. But river is the bed and the water together; it's the figure and ground together.

This sacred feminine function is the *active principle of wholeness*, a figure–ground dynamism that exposes this invisible half, the one that gives context and meaning to that which it gently uplifts and holds. And in this potentiated space, both are recognized, integrated, and often transformed.

Many nursing actions take place against a background invisible to the eye not attuned to its subtle presence. To be truly conscious of the essence of the total experience is to continually seek the invisible half of wholeness. The *essence* of nursing practice uncovers more information about what is transpiring within the dynamic nature of figure–ground relationship; the person and their whole being (physical situation, relationships, desires, disappointments, expectations, life demands, etc.) become visible to both the nurse and themselves. For those who truly offer a healing presence, figure–ground awareness is the key to helping the person identify and unite the human and the spiritual.

As we revisit the archetypal feminine, mythical stories hold a very different image from what is portrayed in our current reality of the feminine. From the Grail legends, Robert Sardello notes (Sussman, 1995):

> The women of the Grail are representatives of the soul which houses qualities necessary for transforming the self, for realizing that true individuality lies in coming to know ourselves as human spiritual beings. None, absolutely none, of the women figures of the Grail are passive; they are all receptive, and a totally new, active sense of the quality of radical receptivity is recognized.

At this critical juncture for humankind, individuals are remembering these dynamic archetypal feminine qualities, and this is marshalling a new consciousness in the larger healing field. Both women and men are increasingly working with the feminine energies that interact directly with cycle, rhythm, resonance, reciprocity, and right relationship with all things, including "mother" earth.

Discoveries in neuroscience are exploring the capacities of the "new brain," the neo-cortex, which demonstrates capacity for cooperation, problem solving, ethical behavior, and compassion (Villoldo, 2010). Simultaneously, the growing movement toward integral medicine is a spiritual revolution regarding what we can become as *human spiritual beings*. The essence of healing feminine energy promotes an instinct for cooperation and an embracing of diversity in its many dynamic forms. Moving into a place of prominence, it renews us while healing the communities to which we belong. Its open and honoring language fosters a sense of the possible, filling us with hope and the optimism to move forward.

Respect is the hallmark of this radically receptive field. Bordering on reverence, it is a simple personal respect for the patient, for colleagues, and for the self. It is also an impersonal awareness at a deeper level, a sensing that we share space on a sacred healing journey with everything in the universe. A Course in Miracles states that "we heal a brother by recognizing his worth." As we bear witness for another, respecting and honoring what is observed, we provide the catalyst for their transformation and our own.

As the feminine energy is remembered, embraced, and once again consciously used in integral medicine, the outcome is nothing less than profound. The balancing of the masculine and feminine is a transforming work that is birthing a new world order. We are moving from an era guided by the Declaration of Independence where models of autonomy and power reigned supreme. Unfolding discoveries in science and art continue to reveal a deeper theme of cooperation and co-creation running through every aspect of life. We have come to realize that each of us *is* the earth, the air, the sun, and a deeply connected part of one another. Thus, our emerging new worldview holds the promise of the birth of the Declaration of *Inter*dependence (Suzuki, 2002).

Worldview—Individual Perspective on How Life Works

Humanity in every era has struggled with two deep questions: How does the world work, and what motivates life within it? An existence lived on the prairie sees things in nature metaphors, whereas an inner city view is more concrete. Our interaction with all aspects of our world is guided by how we experience and view that world. Those with a partial view see the undoing of our "old story" and feel despair when examining "what is" from a limited viewpoint. Cynical vision leads us to see evidence of imperfection, often resulting in a sense of judgment against the efforts undertaken by others to navigate into the "new story."

Soulful eyes, however, see a larger, more holistic, and more realistic picture. Subtle vision penetrates the materialism and reductionism of our times, noting that while old economic and political structures are breaking down, a new order is also emerging. By reaching into fresh scientific evidence while also relating to historical patterns, we gain insight into humanity's continual unfolding toward a higher order (Rifkin, 2009). From this vantage point, we see the larger context without overlooking the details of the present moment. This perspective facilitates a tough optimism coupled with practical expectancy within the chaotic unfolding of our times. A sense of the optimism and hope, rather than despair and hopelessness, is fostered.

Nurses are quintessential knowledge workers; discovery and co-creation are the tools of our trade. Learning is our human birthright. We are born with the innate ability to imagine, wonder, invent, and explore our way into unknown territory, some of which holds paradoxical and perplexing questions (Vaill, 1996). From our first breath, we observe and sense, take things apart and put them back together again, and wonder about the vastness of the universe and our place within it. The starting point of this awareness is awe and wonder. As much as we are an independent entity in the universe, we are also a partner with it. We are both thrilled and perplexed by our human condition. And in our irrepressible pursuit toward understanding, we create our world.

Many of us as individuals, and especially our large social institutions, still subscribe to an outdated worldview that is inadequate to deal with the larger issues of our changing reality. New concepts in physics have shifted our understanding of the universe from the mechanistic and linear worldview of Descartes and Newton to the holistic and interconnected ecological view fostered by discoveries in quantum physics, cellular biology, and neuroscience (Rasha, 2006). A gift of our profession is access to advances in science and technology, which enable us to observe emerging patterns and structures within the universe, giving us a new story of the natural world. Web-based social networks are mirrored in the globalization of business and finance, redefining relationships and exchange. Those unfamiliar with this new way of connecting and learning are limited in being able to fully see, integrate, and appreciate the emerging story of unity and wholeness, reciprocity, interdependence, and co-creation within the unifying web of life (Capra, 1996).

Just as the mechanical model of the universe is being dismantled, so is the disconnected model of our mind–brain–body system (Marshall, 2005). Your own unique perception shapes your reality. By examining the emerging networks of order within the ecological and human worlds, you can begin to recognize and experience the magnificently complex, pattern-seeking, living network of self-adjusting neuronal connections of your own mind/brain. Research is discovering that your thoughts have a powerful role in shaping your mind and brain, literally changing the physical structure of the brain. Human intelligence is not a fragmented and independent process but rather a biological and social one.

Feelings and emotions have been identified as the guiding force for the process of active engagement underlying the construction of knowledge and meaning. Meaning is created as we match new learning with existing patterns, developing new networks of understanding in ever enlarging and encompassing circles. As this awareness is shifting, so is our model for nursing practice.

SCIENCE/ART/PRESENCE: THE TRIAD OF COMPASSIONATE CARE

All health professions are being redefined as this new epoch unfolds. Nursing has traditionally been viewed as an art and a science. Our theories, curriculum, and practice models reflect this framework. Florence Nightingale observed that (Calabria & Macrae, 1994)

> Along with our science, Nursing is an art, and if it is to be made an art, it requires as exclusive a devotion, as hard a preparation as any painter's or sculptor's work; for what is the having to do with dead canvas or cold marble, compared to having to do with the living body, the temple of God's spirit. It is one of the Fine Arts; I had almost said the finest of the Fine Arts.

Careful examination on her reflection reveals a third principle: active receptivity—the feminine spirit that permeates the art and science of our profession. This is the essence of nursing: a healing presence.

As we come to understand this implicit dimension of nursing, we begin to comprehend the profession's three-fold framework: science, art and, presence. When all three domains are present in the nurse–person relationship, a healing gestalt occurs.

Science: Nurses Are Scientists—Professional nursing is founded on a body of knowledge derived from science and research. Measured evidence forms a theoretical framework of the external physical world as the foundation, the object, or focus of our clinical practice. This is the *"evaluator aspect"* of nursing, which comes from the *realm of concrete analytic thought*. Facts, data, and logic guide our practice through evidence-based protocols and standards that point our observations and choices toward predetermined outcomes.

Art: Nurses Are Artists—Experience-based mastery leads to subtle pattern recognition from multiple perspectives, the field or ground of our practice. This *"interpreter aspect"* of nursing is from the *realm of abstract perceptive thought*. Intuition and active awareness of the understated fosters discernment and pattern recognition, which then guides synthesis of unrelated parts into a larger whole. Individualized personal care that supports the interior world of the patient is thus created.

Essence: Nurses Are a Healing Presence—An authentic and patient presence creates a space of *active receptivity* for the person (and their family) that potentiates their own inner resources. The feminine healing function of the *"witness aspect"* of nursing comes from the *realm of no mind: pure consciousness.* Guided by the intent to support what is in the highest good for the person and family, we create an empty space of open, nonjudging expectancy, which allows individuals to connect with their inner wisdom and innate power to heal. As we trust in the other to grow and ourselves to care, we have the courage to go into the unknown together.

Because there is simultaneous attention to the exterior world, the inner world, and the unmanifest Now, the soul is also invited to participate. When we include the numinous in our shared space, transformative insight and energy emerge, enlarging the experience for all. And in that shared exchange, each becomes more. Carl Rogers (1980) observed that, "The degree to which I can create relationships which facilitate the growth of others as separate persons is a measure of the growth I have achieved in myself."

Although nurses bring science, art, and presence to the individual and family, nursing also serves as the heart and soul, the primary surveillance system for the health of society. Because of this fact, a crisis of major proportion is imminent. While political, economic, and environmental issues challenge society, the increasing global shortage of nurses offers one of the greatest hazards to the health and well-being of humankind.

Medical practices vary in different parts of the world, depending on the tools and healing models of the culture. Nursing, on the other hand, is a universal phenomenon. Daily, and nightly, in every part of the world, millions of nurses stand alongside people in need, helping them with maintenance of functional activities of daily living such as mobility, elimination, and pain management. Nurses also assist those who are well in maintaining their health status through educating the public about adequate nutrition and exercise as well as the power of good mental health practices. Finally, and most importantly, nurses also accompany people in their journey toward a peaceful death, supporting families and loved ones in the process. Helping individuals, families, and society manage their inevitable health challenges, while finding meaning in the illness event, is at the core of what it means to be a nurse.

Nursing, as a global community, is in a unique position as midwife to help birth the "new story" for humanity. The Lakota Sioux say that "when the Grandmothers speak (the sacred feminine) the world will heal." For this time in history, we have been preparing. Work of this magnitude must utilize all our resources available to creatively practice the science, art, and essence of nursing.

Science—The Foundation of Knowledge That Guides Our Practice

Today we stand on the threshold of a revolution as daring as Einstein's discovery of relativity. On the frontier of science, new ideas are emerging that challenge everything we have come to believe about the world and how it works. Discoveries are being made that demonstrate what philosophies and religions have held as true: humanity is more extraordinary than a mere physical machine that lives in a self-determined world. Through a dynamic quantum field, we are ever changing and deeply connected to *all that is.*

Scientists in various disciplines have been carrying out well-designed experiments whose results transcend the beliefs of current biology and physics. At the core, what they have uncovered is the fact that we are not a collection of chemical reactions but rather an energetic charge. All living things are a coalescence of energy emerging from a universal, pulsating energy field connected to every other thing in the universe. This potent field is responsible for the highest functions of our mind. As an information source, it guides the growth and development of our bodies. It influences our brain, our heart, and our memory. As radical as it may seem, the Universal Zero Point Field, rather than genes or germs, determines whether we are healthy or ill. It is, in the end, the force that must be tapped in order to heal (McTaggart, 2002).

Conventional science is grounded in the idea that matter is the building block of all things. Life, mind, and awareness are held to be secondary phenomenon of matter. In the prevailing science, elementary particles make atoms, atoms make molecules, molecules make cells including neurons, neurons make the brain, and the brain makes awareness. The "theory of causation" holds that the interactions between the elementary particles create various forms of matter, moving from smaller to larger objects in predictable fashion. Dualistic "either-or" and "cause-effect" thinking has been the hallmark of reason for more than 400 years.

Quantum physics uncovers a reality more dynamic and connected than that put forward by conventional science. Upon examining this evolving research, one learns that several discoveries have already determined that rather than a universe of static certainty, matter at the most fundamental level, and the world which it builds, is uncertain and unpredictable, a state of pure potential and infinite possibility (Hollick, 2006). Subatomic particles are not seen as solid objects but rather as vibrating and indeterminate packets of energy that cannot be precisely quantified or controlled. These energy packets can take on the quality of a particle and either stay confined in a small space, spread over a large region of space time in wavelike fashion, or do both simultaneously, that is, test out all possible new electron orbits at once.

Werner Heisenberg, an architect of quantum theory, established the Uncertainty Principle, which demonstrates that nothing is certain: there are no definite locations for these quantum energy packets only a likelihood or a probability that they may settle into a specified pattern. Based on this finding, cause-and-effect relationships no longer exist at the subatomic level, for stable looking atoms suddenly elect to transfer from one energy state to another in an unpredictable leap (Heisenberg, 1971). Suddenly, amidst the known and expected, we are aware of the startling and unpredictable "quantum leap" activity surrounding us. An unsettling quickening of activity and possibility is now the new hallmark of our times.

Quantum physics demonstrates that subatomic particles have a capacity for cooperation. They not only get in synch but are also highly interlinked by bands of common electromagnetic fields so they can communicate with each other, like multiple tuning forks resonating together. As they get into phase together, they begin to act like one giant subatomic particle, creating a single large wave. What is done to one then affects the whole. Coherence establishes communication and high levels of quantum order (Bohm & Hiley, 1993).

Traditional science defines relationship by geographic proximity. Now the concept of nonlocality shatters this foundational principle of conventional physics. Once in contact with another, a quantum entity such as an electron retains a connection even when separated by time and space. Actions of one will continue to influence the actions of the other, no matter how far they are separated by time or distance (Nadeau & Kafatos, 2002). This phenomenon explains the power of prayer and meaningful relationships in the healing experience.

One of the most essential ingredients of this interconnected universal web of energy is the impact on the awareness of the person observing it. In classic physics, an experimenter is considered separate and apart from the experiment. The scientist is simply an impartial observer in the process. In contrast, quantum physics reveals that the state of all possibility is collapsed into a set entity when it is observed or measured. There is a strong relationship between the observer and the observed. In fact, the observer creates the observed object (Pribram, 1991). "In other words, actual "things" that are different from us, or distinct in themselves, enter consciousness by virtue of our perception and the sensibility that informs perception."

Classic laws of science have been very useful for describing fundamental properties of motion such as locomotion and respiration and for explaining how basic body processes such as digestion and sensory input operate. But classic physics and biology have been unable to explain fundamental issues such as how we think, why arms and legs develop differently, how cells cure themselves of cancer, and how we know what we know. The emerging model of science begins to uncover a deeper reality, one that more fully explains the mysteries of the universe and our place within it (Villoldo, 2008).

Art—The Intuitive Skill of Pattern Recognition

Both art and science are unique forms of language describing the same reality, with art leading the way. Artists and authors, especially those writing science fiction, depict what is about to be born in society. Art begins with a vision. It is preverbal in nature and precedes abstract ideas as well as the words and actions that describe and explore them. Visionary artists (nurses) alert others that a shift is about to occur because their vision is a particular prescience. They mysteriously incorporate into their work features of a physical description that science later discovers or proves (Shlain, 1991).

Nurses walk between two worlds, the material world of a scientist and the creative world of an artist. Our craft depends on a well-developed sense of aesthetics: if it does not "look right," it is not functioning properly. The intuitive capacity of the nurse is the heart of the sentinel function at the bedside, which notes a subtle shift heralding a potential crisis. Early identification assures intervention with the least amount of effort to restore balance.

Physicians most trust the nurse who lives in the realm of the aesthetic subtle. This nurse will call and report, "All vital signs are normal, but something is wrong; come now!" This nurse is sensing a faint shift in pattern that lies below the surface of articulation or measurement. Intuition and an appreciation for symmetry are guardians in the understated background of surveillance. Well developed, they are the gift a master practitioner brings to her or his profession.

Nurses rely heavily on the intuitive visual–spatial right hemisphere of their brain. At the same time, scientific rigor builds a deep repository of facts and data that figure into the logic and reason emanating from the left hemisphere. As a scientist, they break the nature of things into discrete parts to analyze their relationships in reductionistic fashion. As an artist, nurses synthesize varying aspects of the person's present state through stories, symbols, and metaphors to explore emotions and generate new perspectives. There is considerable crossover in the skills and techniques used in both functions. Shuttling between the two spheres with grace, the *active intelligence* of the nurse integrates the complimentary function of both sides into a larger whole.

Essence—The Authentic Healing Presence of the Nurse

Systems of art and science are modified over time, creating and organizing new knowledge in terms of, and in response to, a specific set of issues or problems. The overarching evolutionary progress of humanity has always been toward higher order. In the past 300 years we have made vast strides in the worlds of art and science, learning to harness and distribute energy while creating new forms of machines, materials, and beauty. What has been slower in development is the subjective psycho/social/spiritual side of humanity. Our power to manipulate and control the "outside" world has advanced greatly, but we have not made similar advances in understanding our own behavior and our "inner" experience.

Current challenges facing society in general, and health care in particular, are pressing for a new way to comprehend and enhance the "inner world" of humankind. The lack of advances in understanding human behavior and inner experience has prevented us from solving pressing issues such as war, the world population explosion, and the poisoning of our planet. On a personal scale, we are experiencing the growth of lifestyle-related chronic illness at all ages and stages of the life continuum. Depression, mental illness, addiction, and obesity point to a culture deeply in search of meaning as old forms and processes fall away.

Conventional healing efforts have been focused into the past, trying to unearth the origins of patterns that do not serve us well. Health care professionals have traditionally helped people who are suffering to focus on contextual issues within their lives: family, career, social, and economic issues. However, the indigenous perspective in healing offers us a new and transformative approach to illness and crisis. Stepping out of our life situation—becoming witness—opens up the present moment, a larger context where resolution resides.

When our mind is filled with problems, there is no room for anything new to enter, no room for a solution. Whenever we can create some space, we will find the life that exists underneath the situation, the life that is our birthright. In most people's normal state of awareness, they identify with their thought processes, reactions, desires, and aversions. Run by the ego, they are in a continuous low level of unease, discontent, boredom, or nervousness—a constant background static. This keeps them unaware and out of touch with the "being" side of their nature. They live in a state of inner pollution.

Becoming conscious occurs when we truly step into the moment. As we learn to witness our own thoughts and emotions, rather than being driven by them, we become surprised at the freedom in the world. Anything unconscious becomes conscious as we turn our focus toward it, and the light of our presence shines more brightly.

Nurses have long observed the spiritual dimension of healing, but little of this is captured in the medical record. Yet, we intuitively recognize that the spiritual side of human nature is an essential aspect of the healing process.

> There is a force that is unfathomable, omnipresent, unnamable and omniscient. This intelligent and loving force stands behind and guides the evolution of physical manifestation. Spirituality is the label used to describe what occurs when we connect with this source.
>
> *Unknown Teacher*

The source of spirituality emerges from many names: Organizing Wisdom, Great Spirit, Creator, Christ Within, Atman, God, The Field, The Universal, The One. We connect to this source automatically and often when least expected. Understanding spiritual truth occurs as we remove blocks to its recognition. Just as opening the blinds in a dark room allows the sunlight to pour in, opening to our innate spiritual nature invites the new and unexpected to emerge. In their compelling book, *The Spirituality of Imperfection*, Kurtz and Ketcham observed (Kurtz & Ketcham, 2002):

> Spirituality points, always, beyond: beyond the ordinary, beyond possession, beyond the narrow confines of self, and—above all— beyond expectation. Because the "spiritual" is beyond control, it is never exactly what we expect.

Tapping into the deeper levels of being where our true innate intelligence resides requires bringing the spiritual dimension into the healing process. As we integrate our inner rhythms into our life, we begin to experience a flowing interconnectedness around us, which eventually includes the entire human and planetary family. Holistic physician Hogben notes (Chopra, 1989):

> Healing may be defined as a miraculous unfolding of consciousness for one's being in the world. We learn who we are, what and who really matter to us, how to express ourselves fully and openly. Ultimately the healing journey leads to an intimate union with the One through the experience of the flow of Spirit within. It is a slow, arduous passage, unique for each individual, filled with danger and risk, triumph and joy, and finally, peace, trust, awe, reverence, love and compassion.

Healing goes beyond dealing with a health problem or crisis. It touches every aspect of life, facilitating a continuous movement toward wholeness and peace. In order to support the healing of others, we must also be on the path ourselves. Therefore, nurse and patient are partners in this expansive journey toward wholeness.

A health challenge creates an opening in time and space from which flow the inner feelings, hopes, intentions, expectations, memories, pain, and decisions that give depth and context to the person suffering. At this "edge of existence" lie the opportunity and the invitation to become more fully who we are.

Supporting the deeper soul work of healing, nurses assist people with physical and emotional challenges and fears in more authentic fashion. No longer do we analyze the event or look to the past or present circumstances for explanations. No longer do we foster resistance to weaknesses or deep feelings of sadness with "will power" or "discipline." Instead, we help the person stay with their feelings and learn to observe them without reaction, description, or interpretation. In that open state, a relationship is created between the person and their true qualities or essence, opening up the possibility for real transformation and growth.

SELF-KNOWLEDGE: THE KEY TO HEALING PRESENCE

To offer a safe and open space for deep self-reflection, we must know our own authentic self. This may involve the process of seeing where we came from just so we can let it go and move forward. A lovely paradox is found: although fear is always directed toward the future, that which haunts us—that which is creating the fear—is derived from the past. The call to authenticity is not a call to perfection; that is an impossible goal.

> Once a student of Carl Rogers, noted psychologist and founder of a "person-centered approach to life," asked this noted therapist a question; "How is it that every time I see you with a patient, any patient, they immediately open up to you with such candor?" Dr. Rogers replied, "Before I go into any room, I remind myself that I am not perfect. I am human. Therefore, I am capable of any thought/emotion/act that has ever been had. Being perfect is not enough. I am called to be human, and in that space I am one with all I meet. (Rogers, 1980)."

Socrates encouraged us to "know ourselves." Knowing our own self in this deep sense includes the past as well as our true potential, which represents the future. As we move toward truly knowing our self and our inherent qualities, we are released from being haunted by the past, which limits our freedom to "be." Our true essence emerges, creating space for others to more fully touch their own.

Socrates was inviting us to have a relationship with ourselves, because then no one can haunt us or claim responsibility for who we are. True freedom comes through knowing our self, and *this does not require a need to change anything*. All that is needed is to see what has been, without reacting to it in any way. In so doing, we put an end to the story; we transcend patterns and expectations of our history to become the qualities, the real essence, of our being. This is wholeness. And, once acquired in our life, we can hold space for others to find their own way home.

> Give us grace, O God, to dare to do the deed which we well know cries to be done. Let us not hesitate because of ease, or the words of (people's) mouths,
> or our own lives. Mighty causes are calling us—the freeing of women,
> the training of children, the putting down of hate and murder and poverty—
> all these and more. But they call with voices that mean work and sacrifice and death. May we find a way to meet the task.
>
> W. E. B. Du Bois

BIBLIOGRAPHY

Bohm, D., & Hiley, B. (1993). *The undivided universe: An ontological interpretation of quantum theory*. New York, NY: Routledge.

Brisken, A. (2005). *Rishi*. Oakland, CA: Unpublished manuscript.

Calabria, M. D., & Macrae, J. A. (1994). *Suggestions for thought by florence Nightingale: Selections and commentaries* (p. 120). Philadelphia, PA: University of Philadelphia Press.

Capra, F. (1996). *The web of life: A new scientific understanding of living systems*. New York, NY: Doubleday Dell Publishing Group.

Chopra, D. (1989). *Quantum healing* (pp. 48–49). New York, NY: Bantam Books.

Heisenberg, W. (1971). *Physics and beyond*. New York, NY: Harper & Row.

Hollick, M. (2006). *The science of oneness: A worldview for the twenty-first century*. New York, NY: Maple Vail Press.

Kurtz, E., & Ketcham, K. (2002). *The spirituality of imperfection: Storytelling and the search for meaning*. New York, NY: Bantam Books.

Marshall, S. (2005). "A decidedly different mind," Shift: At the frontiers of consciousness. *September-November, 2005*(8), 14–17.

McTaggart, L. (2002). *The field*. New York, NY: HarperCollins Publisher.

Nadeau, R., & Kafatos, M. (2002). *The non-local universe: The new physics and matter of the mind*. New York, NY: Oxford University Press.

Pribram, K. H. (1991). *Brain and perception: Holomony and structure in figural processing*. Hillsdale, NJ: Lawrence Ehrlbaum.

Rifkin, J. (2009). *The empathic civilization: The race to global consciousness in a world in crisis*. New York, NY: Penguin Group.

Rogers, C. (1980). *A way of being* (p. 43). Boston: Houghton Mifflin, Company.

Shlain, L. (1991). *Art & physics: Parallel visions in space, time & light*. New York, NY: Simon & Schuster.

Sussman, L. (1995). *Speech of the grail*. New York, NY: Lindisfarne Press.

Suzuki, D. (2002). *The sacred balance: Rediscovering our place in nature*. Vancouver, CA: Graystone Books.

Vaill, P. (1996). *Learning as a way of being*. San Francisco, CA: Jossey-Bass Publishers.

Villoldo, A. (2008). *Measuring the immeasurable: The scientificcxase for spirituality*. Boulder, CO: Sounds True Publishers.

Villoldo, A. (2010). *Illumination*. Carlsbad, CA: Hay House.

CHAPTER 2

A HEALING JOURNEY
BETWEEN TWO CULTURES
AN EXPERIENCE OF WHOLENESS

Healing will happened.
Health is optional.
Wellness is the Balance

Wanigi Waci

During my 40-year nursing career, I have been privileged to sit with patients and families of patients awaiting imminent death. I have had the honor of helping families cope with difficult medical decisions. I have been present with many people in their suffering. However, not one of those many encounters over the years prepared me for a personal experience of healing that changed my worldview forever.

This personal crisis followed a long and difficult pregnancy, multiple surgeries, and a series of medical errors. My daughter Kristi was moved into our home mid-pregnancy when she was put on total bed rest. She, and her colicky newborn son, had been a guest in our home for 8 months now when she returned to the hospital for "one last procedure." Kidney stones had become the latest complication, so a stint had been inserted to assist with stone removal. She had gone into the hospital for kidney function testing and stint removal. Rather than remove the stint, the surgeon had placed a second stint in the other kidney after discovering a total of five stones in both kidneys, which no Western medical treatment could prevent from forming. The resulting pain of stones, stints, and recent surgeries was beyond all pharmaceutical relief. Her breath was short and gasping, her hands clutched the sheets, and her ashen face was drenched with perspiration. But most of all, her disappointment at yet another setback was a devastation she could not endure. It had been almost 9 months since she had been out of bed. Her older son and husband were episodic visitors to our home, and her baby with colic cried most of the day and night. This event took what hope was left within her—she had given up. It was more than I could bear to witness—and there was absolutely nothing I could do for her.

I took her home and put her back to bed one more time. If ever I had wished for the power of the Gods to perform a miracle, this was the moment. Since that was not possible, my sense of inadequacy, frustration, fatigue from 8 months as caregiver, anger, sorrow, and fear raged through my being with a force that transcended every emotion I had ever known. I was shattered and yet held captive by the moment. I had to stay connected. It was like standing with my finger in a live socket, taking the volts of electricity, and not being able to let go. Together, my daughter and I barely endured another seemingly endless night.

The next morning the phone rang. I picked it up expecting it to be my husband. Each day that he was unable to come to Sioux Falls he would call with an update on the status of his beloved daughter. The voice on the other end was not his but rather that of Wanigi Waci, a Lakota Sioux Spiritual Guide.

"Your daughter is very ill."

Hearing the comforting voice of my mentor and friend reduced me to tears and I sobbed, "I know she is, Wanigi Waci, but I have run out of ideas on how to help her."

"If you like, I can bring medicine to her, Jo," he offered.

Little did I know that this offer would take me into another dimension of health and healing, to a place I had never been before, a place that would explain the appearance of the five stones and the meaning they held for the women in my ancestry.

THE CONTEXT OF SUFFERING

I am a scientist, and I am a nurse. I have practiced every form of nursing during my rich and lengthy career: educator/practitioner/regulator/entrepreneur. Each experience deepened my understanding and respect for the discipline, which has been central to my existence since I was 5 years old and "knew" that I wanted to be a nurse. My experiences ranged from bedside nursing in a tertiary care center, to clinic nursing as a physician's assistant in a town of 600 people, to serving as president of the American Organization of Nurse Executives while then President Clinton was working on Health Care Reform in Washington, DC. In all that time, I loved every aspect of the work, the discipline, the health care field. I knew that what we offered was enhancing to the health of society. That is, until the system that I had given my life to started to unravel before my eyes. Each medical error and negative experience encountered by our daughter led to deeper levels of despair at the complexity and challenge facing the industry today. Finally, when she was totally bedridden, and no help was in sight, I quit my job and took her into our home. In that experience—I became a healing presence.

Life had become a blur of activity. Following a complex, bed-ridden pregnancy and an emergency C-section, Kristi's world in bed consisted of hot packs, cold packs, back rubs and foot massage, pain medications every 4 hours, drinking gallons of water, and frequent urination irritated by the presence of stints in both kidneys. Kidney stones were multiplying, and hypertension and an endocrine system shift complicated matters further. Interwoven into daily routine were frequent trips to the medical clinic and hospital for tests, x-rays, CAT scans, and the constant discouraging message of "no change." There were brief periods of rest or quiet, never more than several hours, coupled always, always with the companionship of pain, which demanded its share of attention from us all. Simultaneously there was JJ, a precious but colicky child, trapped by hunger and then hours of cramps and pain half an hour after feedings that would find him crying and screaming for relief. He too would receive hot packs, cold packs, aromatherapy and massage therapy. Our world became one of short rest intervals surrounded with hours of struggle by both mother and child. Interwoven into that scenario was 18-month-old Ethan who wondered what was happening to his world. Days consisted of daycare, a brief visit with a mother who could not even hold him, and then home to bed and nights filled with nightmares and longing. Eugene, her husband, kept one side of his family afloat, while I attempted to buoy up the other. Life became a lesson in endurance.

In the midst of all this, I became acutely aware of several lessons. If one has a declared chronic illness, life is adjusted and accommodations are made. Each trip to the physician found us receiving the same message; "There is no explanation for this continued development of stones and why they are not passing. We must wait and see what the stones will do. Until then, the stints must both remain." The undetermined path and time frame prevented any long-term planning. We attempted to keep "business-as-usual" while responding to the demands of the moment. A sense of unmanageable chaos permeated our lives.

The far greater lesson was one about suffering. I discovered that suffering is a dimension, much like time and space. In the dimension of suffering, time has no relevance. There is no hurrying it in any way. One must learn to slow down to the pace of what is happening and work with the rhythms that it holds. All of life stops when suffering is profound. Focus leaves the external world and moves into an interior space, the place of longing, and the ultimate meaning of existence. It was into this space that Wanigi Waci entered.

LAKOTA WAYS OF HEALING

My relationship with Wanigi Waci began while I was CNO at Sioux Valley Hospital in the mid-1990s as we established policies and procedures for improving care offered to the SD Native American population. It was very formal when we first met, but as time went on a deep and sustained friendship developed. Being invited into some of the rituals and ceremonies of his tribe, I came to appreciate the qualities of his culture and his worldview. A real surprise was the discovery of his world's profound sense of humor and play. It would not be uncommon to leave an Inipi Ceremony with a string of empty cans and bottles tied to the bottom of my car, bouncing merrily all the way home. After a formal meeting, I would be alerted to a clothespin clipped to the back of my suit jacket or coat only by people's chuckles as I walked by. Once after a strategic planning session, I drove away from the meeting with an inflated rubber glove tied to the grill of my car. It wildly waved at me and all that passed by as I drove home.

Wanigi Waci was quick of wit and would always have something to say about a comment made. Once I sent an e-mail about being in a "pickle," in a difficult situation. His response was

From: WW (ww@usd.edu)
Sent: Thursday, June 22, 1999 12:15 PM
To: jokerner@virtual.com
Subject: Lela Waste Elo (That's very good!)

Jo, So what's the big dill about the pickle theory??
I'm sorry that wasn't very kosher was it!
Get the cue-, cumbersome huh?
Well, relish the thought. WW

I took Kristi to the clinic for yet another CAT Scan and pain treatment session. When the 4 hours were up, I returned to the clinic to pick her up. She was quite drugged, but I could see that she had gotten some rest. She said that the pain was less intense but put her finger on a well-known spot on her back, acknowledging a pain that was still very palpable.

As we drove into the driveway I saw a car—Wanigi Waci was waiting. I helped Kristi into the house as he sat by the picnic table on the patio, working with some branches and leaves. After putting her to bed, I went outside and he looked at me so compassionately I almost wept.

"Jo, what are you thinking?" he enquired. I quickly responded in panic, "We have been going through this for months now, and she continues to deteriorate and her pain is relentless.

"Kristi is having very deep and intense pain," he noted. "I have brought her the medicine." He then proceeded to sort through various herbs, leaves, and small twigs. He cut the twigs into tiny pieces, gently and with deep reverence. We sat in silence as I watched him make his preparations. Then he tied the various sorted piles into different colored cloths. He wrote a number on the tie of each one, indicating the order in which they should be taken, and we carried the finished products into the house.

He requested a kettle to cook up a broth of tea for Kristi to drink. He showed me how to smudge myself, Kristi, the work area, all as a prayerful way of acknowledging the healing power of the plants while giving "Wopela"—thanks—to the Creator for these healing gifts. We stood in silence as I watched the small twigs dancing in the boiling water. Suddenly the pot became effervescent, similar to a glass of Alka Seltzer when the tablets fizz. When it was finished, I took a cup of the tea into Kristi's room and told her this was for her pain.

I went back to the kitchen where Wanigi Waci sat at the table. He began to explain. "Jo, in your people's way you make artificial medicine, and it is about your wisdom. You design one medicine to treat the heart, another to treat the lungs, and so on. In our way we always work with natural things. Each thing living has its own intelligence, we do not tell it what to do or where to go. You ask, "How do you know which herb treats which disorder since you classify things?" In our way, we simply trust and respect the innate wisdom of the plant to know where to go and what to do."

He went on, "This medicine is for Kristi only. If you were to take it there would be no effect. My respect for nature and all things is from the heart; it is total. I have such deep respect for natural things that when I speak to them they can hear and recognize my voice. I walked for miles on the reservation where the natural remedies grow and asked, "Which of you would be willing to give your life to heal Kristi?" One by one they would signal to me that they were willing. And so, these plants are here for your daughter. When she takes them, they will know what part of her body needs something and go directly to that place. There they will work with her on the DNA level. She will heal deeply, and completely, in that area. When she dies, her body will return to the Earth Mother, and the wisdom gained from the interchange between the herbs and Kristi will be given back to the earth to recycle in another lifetime for other healing work. Nothing is ever lost, all is retained in the great Circle of Life."

As he was finishing that comment we were both startled to see Kristi standing at the door of the kitchen. I looked up and was stunned by what I saw! For 9 months she had been dealing with deep pain, which had turned her face into a taut mask of suffering. Here Kristi stood, the soft and familiar face of my beloved child visible for the first time in so long.

She was radiant and smiling as she quietly declared "Mom, I have no pain!"

Kristi went on to describe her puzzlement. "When I was at the clinic they were very nice to me. The medicine made me sleepy, and the pain got less severe. But there was always, always this spot (and she referenced the back where her left kidney resides) that aches. It has never stopped, until right now. It's almost as if this medicine knew where to go!" I looked at Wanigi Waci, and he smiled broadly.

THE MEDICINE MAN

Several more months went by with no real change in conditions. By now our fatigue level had led to despair and a sense of help-lessness uncommon to either of us. Suddenly, the phone rang again. Wanigi Waci called to tell me that Kristi's health was not improving, and that if we wished, he would arrange for us to meet with the Medicine Man on a nearby reservation. By now Kristi was very weak, her energy gone, and a sense of subtle despair had set in because the pain was so unrelenting. When I shared Wanigi Waci's offer with her, she immediately lit up. She had such deep respect for him and had experienced the power of his presence before, so she quickly and enthusiastically agreed.

A Wase Wakpa community elder called to guide me in preparing for the event. Rather than bringing an insurance card, I had to offer prayers and forgiveness, plan a feast of *Wopela* (thanksgiving) for those who would come to support Kristi in ceremony, and obtain give-away gifts for the Medicine Man and his helpers. Asking the Creator for healing is a significant event. It required me to conduct a personal inventory to forgive and seek forgiveness around any ill will or resentments I held before I could participate in a healing ceremony for Kristi. In addition, I gathered up all the needed materials and sat through the night in prayerful preparation, making 401 prayer ties and 6 spirit flags as an offering to the community and the Great Spirit.

I asked my mother to help Eugene with both JJ and Ethan so that I could take Kristi on this journey. She was getting deep satisfaction from being "needed" and had developed a very special relationship with little JJ. Interestingly, she demonstrated more strength and energy than I had seen for some time. After 4 days of preparation, all was gathered, and early in the morning Kristi and I packed the car and left for the Reservation.

Both Kristi and I were quite apprehensive, not knowing what to expect. I had a colleague who had been invited to a similar ceremony. The Medicine Man saw his cancer and told him that he had a short time left to live and encouraged him to go home and spend quality time with his family. I was not sure I could handle the truth if it was not favorable to Kristi's life and health. However, I also knew that we were at a crossroads and nothing was helping.

The July day was particularly beautiful. I can still see the clear blue sky and the huge white clouds that dotted the horizon. We drove through the Badlands, and the colors on the spires were especially radiant. I felt so alive, so present to the moment. A deep sense of excitement and anticipation surrounded us both. We came to a small creek as directed, drove up the hill, and arrived at the designated site. It consisted of a small white house on the top of a hill with a vista of the Badlands that went on endlessly with no signs of civilization. It was truly stepping into a timeless space, and the beauty and peace of that place stay with me to this day.

Shortly after our arrival, the Elder and his wife drove up. With their help, Kristi and I set up a portable table, placing on it a small stove to begin preparing the meal. Kristi sat on a camping stool and helped as she could. While we were busy cooking, a summer storm gathered on the horizon. Winds began to blow wildly as the sky got black with boiling clouds. All around us sheets of rain fell so hard that you could hear them roar as they hit the ground. I inhaled their delicious scent. Amazingly, not a drop fell where we were sitting.

Suddenly Kristi cried aloud, "Look Mom!" To our right the storm was raging, while to our left a cloud had parted, allowing a long silver beam of light to shine forth. It created the most incredible double rainbow I have ever seen. The rainbow arched the entire horizon before us. We were awed at its beauty and the promise it held. Many times later, when Kristi was in her darkest hour, she would comment on the beauty and serenity of that moment. Its power carried us both.

As darkness fell on the land, the Medicine Man and a host of people, including several cars of Wasa Wakpe Community members who had driven several hundred miles, began to assemble around the white house. An Inipi Sweat Lodge Ceremony was held for cleansing and preparation for the Healing Ceremony. Because Kristi was so weak, she and I were allowed to stay by the cooking fire and prepare for the feast.

After the Inipi Ceremony was complete, Wanigi Waci and the Elder told me it was time to meet the Medicine Man and tell him why I brought my daughter. What was it that I wanted from the Creator? I had to go alone to make my request; protocol declared that the mother would offer the petition on behalf of the daughter. Kristi was to stay back at the campsite. The Elder gave me his pipe filled with sage and tobacco and escorted me to meet this incredible man.

The Medicine Man and Wanigi Waci were standing in a clearing at the edge of the camp—waiting for us. I looked at my dear friend, Wanigi Waci, who was standing alongside me, guiding me in English, and translating to the Medicine Man in Lakota. A striking Native American male in his mid-forties, he was dressed in his usual style, jeans and a ribbon shirt. His long black hair was tied back, and the large buckle on his belt shone in the light of the early night stars. His beautiful brown eyes, which hold witness to many dimensions simultaneously, were filled with compassion. His hands, gentle while roughened from working with the earth, held the pipe as he offered prayers in the sacred way his voice drops when he addresses the Creator.

I felt safe and cared for as I stood beside my friend while he guided me through the appropriate protocol. I thought, "So this is what a patient feels like when a nurse stands by." I was filled with a great sense of awe for the wonderful essence of a healing presence. I handed the pipe to the Elder who then handed it to the Medicine Man. He asked, "So, what is it you are seeking?"

I looked into his caring eyes and, with tears brimming my own, I said, "For four generations the women in my family have struggled with childbirth. My great grandmother, my grandmother, and my mother lost their mothers in childbirth. My mother and I almost died when she gave birth to me. I lost two children before having the twins. And now, my daughter Kristi is ill. She almost died in her last delivery, and she cannot seem to recover this time. My deepest prayer, if it is the will of the Creator, is that she will be granted health and recovery so that her children will not experience the life of an orphan."

He looked deeply into my face and then my forehead. Suddenly his eyes widened as he recoiled, and I quickly bowed my head. I knew that he had seen something, and it frightened me beyond belief. Later I would learn that he had "seen" my Emotional Body with the memories of the miscarriages I had incurred. He also could sense into my Causal Body, which held the intergenerational memory of my ancestors, witnessing the multigenerational aspects of this issue.

My heart started to pound wildly, and a dark fear crept inside. It was silent for a very long time. Afraid to look up, I assumed that he was praying. He spoke a few words in Lakota, gave back the pipe, and we moved to the white house.

By now it was totally dark outside, and only a few stars were shining through the clouds that covered the moon. Inside the house, the windows were covered tightly so that no light could enter. The food prepared for the feast, as well as special spirit food, was placed in the center of the room.

Then the people filed into the house, sitting in a large circle. Forty to fifty people had come to share in the healing ceremony for Kristi and two others, one of them being Wanigi Waci's own daughter who was also suffering from a kidney disorder. Kristi and the other two individuals were seated directly in front of the Medicine Man, with me placed at Kristi's left side. When all was ready, the doors were closed and a deep darkness wrapped around us.

Once all the people were settled, a quiet fell over the group, and the Medicine Man set up his altar. It was a simple and eloquent altar made of plywood square with four coffee cans, filled with a special material consecrated to the Spirits, standing the four directions. Spirit flags were placed in the containers along with other spiritual objects. The plywood altar was then covered with the prayer ties we had made, ceremonial flags, and other healing symbols he had taken from his medicine bag. After the altar was assembled, he offered prayers.

The Medicine Man asked the same question in front of the group, articulated in Lakota, which Wanigi Waci translated, to me. "Why are you here, and what is it you are seeking?"

The other two people went first, speaking in their beautiful native tongue.

Then Wanigi Waci said, "JoEllen, tell the people why your daughter is here."

Speaking into the darkness that surrounded us, I began with an apology that I could not speak their language. I repeated what I had said to the Medicine Man and thanked them in German, my native tongue, for the gift of sharing their healing ceremony with us. Kristi reached over to me in the dark, and we squeezed each other's hand, love flowing between us.

Softly the Medicine Man began to pray. Then the Helpers started to sing and drum piercing songs that were offered to the Creator. Suddenly in the darkness, sparks of light began to flicker high in the air. They were slightly larger than a fire fly and blue in color. The sight of them made my heart leap with joyful recognition. As the prayers, songs, and drumming continued, the spirit flashes increased. Then the Medicine Man asked Kristi and the others to stand. Suddenly, she was surrounded by a vortex of whirling light. A loud rattling sound accompanied the swirling energy, and she was tapped repeatedly at various parts of her body, especially over her left kidney. Later we would be told that total darkness is essential because when the spirits enter they see Kristi's body as a silhouette. Wherever illness or injury exists, it appears as a pinhole with the light flowing through. Spirits are drawn to the light and tap and heal the places that show up in this way. I was struck how the process was really a spiritual CAT scan.

Over and over again this scene repeated itself, and suddenly they were gone. All became quiet except for the sound of the Medicine Man's prayers. He sat in silence, and then the lights were turned on. People from the outer circle were invited to offer prayers or comments. One man shared how he had been deeply depressed over the loss of his father a year earlier. During the ceremony, the father appeared to his son, asking him to put his grief down and use that energy to help the people. It was a profound healing for this man. Many people both in the center and the outer ring of the circle experienced healing in multiple ways.

A dish of spirit food was prepared as a thank you offering. The young men served the people. After the feast, give away gifts were offered, and the ceremony ended. It was well past midnight when we exited back into the night. The stars were now out with all their brilliance. Wanigi Waci asked Kristi and me to join him with the Medicine Man. We walked outside. My legs felt like rubber. I could hardly catch my breath, and I was so frightened by what I would hear.

Slowly he began his explanation of our story. "Kristi and Jo, you two come from a wonderful family, a family with a heritage of many good things. However, it is also a culture that has an oppressive history for the women who live within it. The women of your family lineage who died did so because life was simply too hard for them—they chose to leave it. The two of you agreed before coming to this earth plane to live through this time as a way to heal that deep cultural wound. When you heal, the healing will be extended to all the women of your lineage.

Kristi, you have manifested five stones. In our way a stone is a keeper of the memory. These stones represent the five generations of women who have been plagued by death around childbirth; the stones hold their memory. Your earth body is the only thing you uniquely possess, a gift from the Creator. It is given when you are born, and you leave it when you die."

He addressed Kristi with deep compassion, continuing, "Kristi, for you the lesson is one of trust. In your way faith is the path to trust and healing. Faith requires belief in the intentions and power of another. We have faith that someone will heal us, save us, protect us. That faith rests on experiences that need to be repeated to keep the trust alive. In our way it is not faith but rather "knowing." Once we experience something we simply KNOW, and in that knowing nothing ever needs to be proven again. You have now had an experience and you KNOW. Let that wisdom be sufficient to restore your health; you are already healthy. *You have only to realize it and KNOW it at a deep cellular level, and **health** will be yours.*"

Then he turned to me and said, "When one is oppressed they either turn outward or inward. The women in your lineage turned the oppression inward on themselves, and their bodies were destroyed. The key to healing this intergenerational issue is the notion of forgiveness. *Jo, if you want Kristi and this intergenerational issue to **heal**, you must forgive all male oppression in this world.*"

His words staggered me. I looked at Kristi, whom I loved beyond my own life, and I thought of all the issues around patriarchy I had experienced in so many ways as a child. Images flooded my memory from the church and its male-dominated leadership, metaphors, and language, as a nurse working with predominantly male physicians and administrators in both academic and health care environments. HOW, how could I possibly just move through all those years and transcend the memories and feelings that remained? I was suddenly aware of the heaviness I felt that was not only from my own experience but genetically from the women who had preceded me in the family.

I stood there stunned! WHAT was I to do now? How much easier it would be to give a pill or herb, prepare someone for restful sleep, but to "forgive all male oppression?" Then in a flash, I SAW all the ways I have been oppressive in my life. A middle child, fighting with siblings, working parents against each other to get what I wanted. . . .the list was endless. Smiling, Wanigi Waci said to me, "Forgiveness starts with forgiving yourself."

In that moment, I thought of the time he addressed a gathering of nurse executives at the National Center for Nursing Leadership. This incredibly compassionate Native American, whose whole history is laced with oppression, stood up in the group and said. "The world is hard for women, for female energy, for the Earth Mother. I would like to extend an apology to you for all the ways that my gender has hurt you. Reconciliation brings a future. Retribution brings an end". In that sincere apology from Wanigi Waci, many past wounds were healed for everyone present.

Watching me intently now, he saw that I "got it," and we both laughed. I realized I could/must start to forgive myself for all the ways I have caused another to suffer if I wanted good things for someone else. Not to be perfect; to be human is the assignment of the day! Suddenly, being human felt free and light-hearted, and a deep compassion for myself and all other beings flooded me with a warmth and deep peace. My relief was so profound I thought for a moment that I would pass out.

With deep gratitude, we profoundly thanked both men and walked away. We got into the car and drove to a small hotel so Kristi could get some sleep. It was 3 A.M. when we crawled into bed totally exhausted and amazed by what had just transpired. Wanigi Waci stayed up all night and prayed for the people—and for Kristi.

The ride home the following morning was an unusual one. We tried to discuss what had happened. Kristi was so confounded by what she had experienced, she was unable to make any sense of it. Being more detached, and having experienced many of the ceremonies of the community, I had a different perspective of it. However, we both agreed that something very sacred had occurred but that to share details with the rest of the family would be most difficult because they had not experienced it. And more honestly, we could not articulate what we had experienced because we weren't able to explain it using our Western/religious worldview. We realized that both healing and integration of a new way of knowing would take some time.

MOTHER NATURE MOVES

Several weeks later as I drove past my favorite oak tree in the front yard, the one with the swing attached for the grandchildren, I thought I noticed something unusual at the top of the tree. To my dismay, the tree appeared to be dying. The top third of the tree was withered, all of the leaves dead. "WOW!" I thought to myself.

"It was perfectly healthy when I left 5 days ago, what could be happening?" I quickly called the gardener (who had become a true friend). He appeared the next day. By then, two-thirds of the tree was dead. He shared my concern and gently snipped a small branch off the tree. With concern, he noted that the tree appeared to have a disease that would not only destroy the tree but most possibly ALL of the oak trees in the area.

Heartsick, I asked what I could do. "This is a very contagious disease," he said. "If it was spring and the sap was running up into the trees it would not be so devastating. However, it is the fall, and the sap is returning to the roots. This area's entire forest of oaks has a deeply entwined root system. The only thing we might do is cut a trench three feet deep alongside this bank of trees, but there is no guarantee that any of them will survive."

He then called the County Extension Agent to come and survey the site for this disease, knowing it could well have implications for the entire region.

By the third morning, the entire tree was dead, and a few of the neighboring trees began to exhibit dead branches. I wept at the loss of my beloved tree. It held so many happy memories with the grandchildren. Dennis and I have a special love for trees. Throughout the years, we have planted hundreds of trees in shelterbelts for the animals on the farm. Trees were like a second family to us.

As I was pondering what to do, Wanigi Waci called. We discussed the issues of the day, and then I said, "Wanigi Waci, I do not mean to complain, but my trees, my precious trees, are dying. WHAT can I do about it?"

He was silent a moment and then asked why it was so troubling. "Are you worried about the economic value of your land if the trees die?"

Quickly I could respond, "No, I am just feeling such a deep loss. I love those trees."

Wanigi Waci talked about our Western view of control, how when things didn't go the way we wanted we would step in and control them. Maybe the trees had completed their life cycle and it was time to dematerialize so they could continue their evolutionary journey. One choice would be to dig the trenches, call in the troops, and try to stop further destruction. A second way would be to honor the natural flow of things, both in nature and our own life. Had I not just gone through a deep life experience that ended some things so that new ones could emerge? By doing so, I was giving the trees permission to evolve also. He suggested that trees are living things, and if I chose to honor nature's rhythms, a ceremony of appreciation would be in order.

Later that day I received the following response to an e-mail I sent enquiring about such a ceremony:

> From: WW (ww@usd.edu)
> Sent: Wednesday, August 30, 2000 9:23 AM
> To: jkoerner@virtual.com
> Subject: Trees
>
> Prayers and their meanings are in direct proportion to heart intent. (Jo to tree), "Why are you leaving? Why are you dying?" (Tree to Jo), "We are still here and will continue to hold the resonance in the immaterial for fifty years or more. . . .or less as we have in the material world. Time is a construct of your will. The real question is, "Jo human, why are you leaving us in your mind? Expand your consciousness and it will all work out in the end, or was it the beginning? Us trees tend to get confused some- times about what an end and a beginning are, silly of us!"
> Do a sacred ceremony; it is essential to manifesting meaning in the space-time of understanding things we hold as real. Test the soil, find the compatibilities, and replant accordingly. . . . . AND have fun!!!

I thought much about the issue of control versus flow and real- ized that in some ways members of my family had been disturbed by the way Kristi and I wove Indigenous and Western healing together. Had we stayed only in the Western traditions, I would not have come to know the spiritual meanings of this illness. What transpired would have been very different. If I had claimed the right to grow, change, and evolve, so should that right be extended to every other living thing. I went outside and performed a small sacred ceremony of gratitude to the tree and the entire little forest that surrounds our place.

The next morning I awoke early, eager to see what was hap- pening to the trees. To my total amazement, I could not see out. Darkness covered the entire kitchen window. Upon closer exami- nation, I saw that it was covered with thousands of tiny winged creatures that were crawling and swarming on the glass. I ran to the door, and as I threw it open, hundreds flew into the house. Quickly I slammed it shut and stood in total amazement. WHAT was this? I went outside and found the entire south side of the house engulfed with these creatures.

At that moment the phone rang; it was Wanigi Waci. We talked about the things of the day, and then I said once again, "Wanigi Waci, I do not mean to complain, but the most bizarre thing is happening. My house is surrounded with thousands, maybe millions, of small winged creatures that are swarming around. I don't know what to do!"

A light chuckle came from the other end of the phone. "Jo, you live at the edge of an old golf course. Think of all the pesticides and other toxic things sprayed through the years to get the effect of beauty in that space. How many times did excessive watering of the greens lower the water table? Think of the number of ways that nature was manipulated and controlled by man to create the desired effect." In my mind's eye, I could see the "pest control programs" and "watering patterns" that had been such a large part of the history of the place.

Wanigi Waci went on, "You have just gone through a healing at the deep belief level, down at the genetic and ancestral level. EVERYTHING is changing within you. Since everything is interconnected, everything around you also will change. The exterior manifests the interior. All things are seeking new balance, a new center."

I stood affixed, not knowing what to say as the bugs kept swarming in my view.

"You have several choices, just like with the trees. You could control them and call an exterminator who would spray them and suppress them back into control. It would work for awhile at least." I quickly protested saying I knew that was not the answer. However, I could not allow the bugs to totally destroy the very foundation of the house.

Wanigi Waci had an alternative suggestion. "Do you have a place that they could move to, is there a hospitable place for them to live?" Quickly I replied, "Oh yes, we have planted a spot just for 'critters' !" "Well then, why don't you invite them to live there?" was the reply.

I thought for a few moments, and never having spoken to bugs before I started to laugh. "Wanigi Waci, HOW do you invite bugs to another space?" He said, "It's time for you to start using your intuition instead of always seeking answers from me. What do bugs and ants like? They like sweet things. Could you offer them something sweet as an enticement?"

The next thing I knew, I found myself mixing a large bottle of sugar water, and carefully slid out of the house through a side door. I walked the full length of the south side of the house that was teaming with the creatures, pouring a trail of sweet water as I went along. I invited them to relocate to a place that was more hospitable to them, and asked them to please leave the house alone. There was plenty of space for all of us, but we each had a unique place to dwell. I laced the majority of the sweet liquid among the trees and bushes we had intentionally planted for critters.

I went back into the house and busied myself with other things. Several hours later, I returned outside and not a single bug was left. The natural space we had reserved for critters was teaming with little creatures setting up housekeeping. When I returned to the house, I discovered the foundation so badly shifted that there were large cracks in basement walls inside the house. The concrete patio that wrapped around the house had been broken in several places. The house had literally been shifted on its foundation! But I never saw another creature on the side of the house. They had truly moved into another space. And the oaks were strong and healthy with no more sign of disease!

GIVING BACK

Several months later, the phone rang again; it was Wanigi Waci inviting me to lunch. As we finished our meal, he said, "Now it is time for you to go on the hill and give back to the great Creator. Kristi lived because of your fervent prayers, and so you must now give something back."

For a very long time, I had wanted to do go on the hill but knew I was not ready for a Vision Quest. The thought of this opportunity was both exciting and terrifying. What if I could not stay on the hill, do without food and water, face fears that would overwhelm me, receive a message that might destroy me? A host of thoughts rushed through my mind, but I heard my calm voice coming from somewhere say, "Thank you for the privilege Wanigi Waci. I am most honored to go on the hill to fast and pray for all the people".

Preparation for a Vision Quest is a major event. I once again made 405 prayer ties along with six spirit flags, but this time the focus and intent of the prayers were different. This time it was about gratitude and surrender—it was preparing me to go back into "The Void."

Four Inipi sweat lodge ceremonies had to be performed as part of the preparation. During the 4 days prior to the Quest, I had a sense of needing to put things in order. I found a strange pattern to the e-mails I was getting and sending. I tried to recall every misdeed and contact people to apologize. Simultaneously, I received a note from a high school classmate, seeking forgiveness for the rude manner in which she had treated me 30 years earlier. Folks appeared out of my distant past with messages and thoughts that were heartwarming or thought provoking. In my dreams, I would see places I had been to and people I knew whom I needed to follow up with a message the next day. By the time the appointed moment arrived, I felt very centered and grateful to be going to a sacred place to say *wopila, Danke Schoen (*thank you) to the great healing Creator. The last message I got on my e-mail system came from Wanigi Waci.

> From: WW (ww@usd.edu)
> Sent: Thursday, August 31, 2000 10:02 AM
> To: jkoerner@virtual.com
> Subject: Ich bin auf der Welt zu allein und doch nicht allein genug
>
> Jo, please answer your CELL phone, God is calling!! For too many
> there has been busy signals or call waiting with 'I'll call you
> back as soon as I'm done" answers. Look within! The macrocosm
> is reflective of the microcosm, therein is the power—Universal
> Consciousness and not just mind power. The first is the total
> essence of the self within all of life throughout eternities. The later
> is the figuring abilities to 'master' this existence! "Simple, but it's
> true, spirits are all around you, but you have to do your part! All
> you have to do is open up your heart" Wopela, Wanigi Waci

I packed up my things and drove to Vermillion. I joined others on the same "quest," setting up a small tent and providing drinks and food for the people who would watch and pray while we fasted on the hill.

A Vision Quest is a time outside of time. Prayerful preparation is essential prior to going on the hill. After we donned our ceremonial dress, we walked in silence to the Inipi Lodge and joined the community gathered. Wanigi Waci took our prayer ties, spirit flags, and all the other spiritual materials that had been prepared at the altar and disappeared down the hill. He was creating individual alters and prayer space at isolated spots on the hill where each of us would experience our Vision Quest alone. The length of time for each individual would be determined by the Spirits. When Wanigi Waci returned, the Ceremony began.

All "Seekers" waited by the fire ring until it was their turn. As each of us individually experienced the initiating ceremony, we were escorted to the hill. An initiating Inipi Ceremony cleanses the body in preparation for going into a sacred space. Wanigi Waci, the singers, and drummers entered first. I was placed at the door of the Lodge, and as community members would enter, they would embrace me, wish me well, and often ask for specific prayers for significant people or events in their life. Then each community member slowly crawled into the low-hanging lodge, with humility, on bended knee.

My helpers (two women of the tribe who had agreed to support me during the Vision Quest) escorted me into the Inipi Sweat Lodge. All of the community members were gathered outside the lodge, and each gave a farewell greeting. Some had special prayers they wanted said for loved ones while on the hill. With all the prayers and good wishes ringing in my ears and my heart, I slowly went into the Lodge for one last prayer session. When it was finished, I was wrapped in the star quilt before leaving. No one was to see my face until I returned from the hill and was cleansed once more in an Inipi Ceremony. For all practical purposes, I was now dead to the physical world.

All I could see was my bare feet as I left the lodge. I felt the strong arms of my two helpers who escorted me down a path to where my prayer circle had been set up by Wanigi Waci. The entire tribal community had left the Lodge to accompany me down the hill, with the sounds of their drumming and chanting as my companion. When they got close to the prayer site, they all turned their backs, and Wanigi Waci took me the rest of the way to my circle. I stood before him, covered with the blanket. Then he gently removed, it and gave me instructions for the time I was to be on the hill.

As he left he smiled and said, "Jo, LISTEN to the voice of God, and pray, pray hard for the people." And with that he was gone. I was alone on a hillside with a star quilt, matches, and a sleeping bag. The experience that unfolded and interpretations from Wanigi Waci are expressed fully in the book (Koerner, 2003, pp. 162–180).

After an intense 48 hour adventure, with unsettling but inspiring visions and experiences, I suddenly heard the drums. I heard the chants. I knew that the people were coming to get us. One by one, they would gather us up and take us home.

My sense of joy knew no bounds! I leaped up with a happiness that fairly bubbled up from deep within. Much as a patient who recovers from cancer, I realized I had another chance to reenter the world and be a more loving and forgiving force within it. Never again would I judge so harshly the ways of anyone, not even myself. We all live out of a cosmology that we inherit from people who are giving us the BEST they can, given what they have experienced and been taught in their own life. Basically, all people have a wonderful core essence, the essence of the Creator. When we keep that in sight, all else is possible.

Quickly I scrambled to my feet, covered myself with the star quilt, moved to a patch of sage, and waited for my escort back to life. I saw the feet of my two helpers who gently put shoes on my feet. They took my arms and guided me back to the waiting caravan of community members who drummed, sang, and chanted as we walked back to the Inipi Lodge. I was escorted inside and was slowly joined by the community. When all were seated, the heated stones were brought in, the door was sealed. In the warmth and darkness of the Lodge, we were allowed to take off the blankets; we had returned home!

Each of us was given a dipper of water, our first in more than 2 days in the relentless South Dakota sun. I wanted it so badly I could just smell and taste it. But, I poured the water on the rocks in memory of the women of my ancestry who had lived such harsh and parched lives. When the second round came, I took the dipper gratefully and sipped it, pouring most of it on my head in a cool baptismal rite.

Then we each were invited to tell our story, sharing what we saw and what we learned on the hill. The community members would make wonderful sounds of encouragement, "ahhhhh, ohhhh, and ho!" as well as shedding tears with us as we wept. The ceremony of storytelling and listening with such sincere intent was a powerful healing in and of itself. After the ceremony was complete, we were escorted outside for a welcoming feast. We thanked the people who had so faithfully offered support during our time on the hill and returned home.

Several weeks after the Vision Quest, several of us offered a Wopila (thank you) feast and a give-away to the Wase Wakpe Community that kept vigil during the Vision Quest. It was a wonderful evening of food and fellowship. We gave presents to each precious community member in deep gratitude for the gifts they had so lovingly bestowed upon us. With tears and a grateful heart, I introduced Kristi, Ethan, and little JJ to those who had not met these people they had prayed for so often. I was able to end with the comment that these children would NOT know the life of an orphan, in part, because of the community's loving support. There were no dry eyes in the room.

I wrote Gene a note of thank you for the unselfish loving gift he and his community had provided. He responded with the following message:

From: WW (ww@usd.edu)
Sent: Tuesday, September of, 2000 10:26 AM
To: jkoerner@virtual.com
Subject: Re: Danke Schoen

Jo,
Wopila for completing your powerful demonstration of love for your daughter, children, grandchildren and fasting soul mates. They gave you purpose and you gave your courage born of love to face fear and dissolve it into what it is, a thought pattern with a lot of value placed upon it by many around you. . . .the Creator is constant and it is only they that are fluctuating between these two extremes. . . . .

Transitions are natural; change is a part of life, everything and everyone is forever evolving at realities in realms of consciousness many times beyond comprehension. Therefore we place ourselves in dream states or vision states to absorb some of this knowledge! The environment around you reflects what is happening within! The more you try to control your yard, focusing in upon the trees, it seems like they are dying! Sadness, alarm, concern for, etc. arises. You have to DO SOMETHING to CONTROL the environment! The more you are attempting to be, someone is alarmed, concerned for, etc. about you seeming to be dying to their reality and you may have to be controlled in some way. All realities are being transformed!

> Are the trees truly dying or transcending a pattern? Are the molecules with the subatomic structures making new partnerships based upon ancient knowingness to rearrange and remanifest in another form of creation? To thy own self be true for at the core of you is the Godness and Goodness of the Original Essence from the Original Source! May the Peace you are be the piece of love someone needs!!
>
> Shalom, Wanigi Waci

A circle of loving and healing had been completed. My sense of relationship had been enlarged through the loving experience of the native community. Nothing was the same, while everything was just as before. The experience of healing at such a deep level gave me a deepened sense of appreciation for all the people whom I had the privilege to witness in their own healing journey during my nursing career. Many dear faces danced through my memory, and I realized that we were all one.

REINTEGRATION

Looking back on the adventure with Kristi, I find that I have learned how to receive as well as give. It is very humbling to seek help and to receive it graciously. That simple act opens up a deeper definition of community. The grace of simple gestures of kindness heals more deeply than the most exalted measures of technology. A balance is needed in all things to acquire the whole. I have returned to my nursing world, which is deeply embedded in science. And yet, I KNOW that it is only part of the equation for healing. Love, intention, spiritual blessing, prayer, all of these are ingredients more powerful than antibiotics and surgery.

This experience has heightened my commitment to the caring agenda in nursing, which is really a call to having an authentic presence that honors the life and values of the person being served. It is my deepest wish that anyone facing a health crisis could have access to not only superb medical care but also the powerful guidance of a healing presence such as Wanigi Waci. By blending the two worlds together, a balanced approach to healing is attained.

Since our experience we continue to find a phenomenon quite common in today's society; repeating patterns of intergenerational health. Repeated requests for help encouraged us to reflect on our experience, and with the help of Wanigi Waci, create an "Intergenerational Guide to Healing" (Koerner, 2003, pp. 187–206). It is with profound respect for your own healing journey that we offer a four-part process that may facilitate your own awareness of intergenerational patterns that may be present in your own family. Such insight can profoundly shift assumptions and influence choices toward a more balanced and healthy life.

One day Wanigi Waci asked me, "How's it going Jo?" I looked at him and said, "You know, I really don't feel like I fit anywhere. It sort of feels like I am a witness to what is happening in life, but not really a part of any world."

He just chuckled and said, "Good! When you 'fit' that means you are molding into someone else's definition of what should be."

"Well then," I prodded, "what is the alternative?"

He looked at me with those large brown eyes twinkling and simply said, "Just BE. When you are BE-ing yourself you will attract other likeminded BE-ings and co-create something new together. Just stay awake, and you will recognize it when it happens."

And that is exactly what is occurring! I continue to meet wonderful people who share similar stories and aspirations. As I move through the world, I am experiencing a heightened awareness of the multidimensionality of the reality in which we live. My profound journey with Kristi and my mother have underscored the fact that life is really a spiritual Odyssey wrapped in a sojourn on this beautiful earth. Everything is deeply connected intergenerationally; what happens to one affects generations that follow. Therefore, we must be good stewards with the life we are given. When we pursue a life dedicated to truth, beauty, and the greater good, the Universe will respond in kind.

BIBLIOGRAPHY

Koerner, J. (2003). *Mother, Heal My Self: An intergenerational healing journey between two worlds.* Santa Rosa, CA: Crestport Press.

Section II

A Healing Presence
The Power of One

*Good listening is ultimately a form
of love. When we listen well we
not only celebrate the other
but we also celebrate ourselves.
By sharing our presence with reverence
we re-enchant and resacralize the world.*

Unknown Teacher

CHAPTER 3

VIBRANT HEALTH
THE ENERGETICS OF DYNAMIC BALANCE

> *The body is the visible soul, and the soul is the invisible body. The body and soul are not divided anywhere, they are parts of each other, they are parts of One Whole.*
>
> Osho

Your body occupies—uniquely—a space in the cosmos; you are a dynamic and self-regulating force in the world! As a vibrant, living field of energy, each being touches and is touched by all-that-is. The continuous universal exchange of energies from the sun and earth flow through every human cell, infusing your body/ mind, enhancing your health and vitality. As our understanding of health as a body/mind/spirit connection to consciousness grows, we begin to "see" the concrete human body and its relationship to the quantum world of energy more clearly.

THE HUMAN BODY RE-VISIONED— AN INTEGRATED FIELD OF ENERGY

To honor preference for differing "ways of knowing," the following information is presented in simplistic and summarized fashion in Tenet Boxes throughout the chapter. For those who seek a more detailed and scientific description of the concept under consideration, a more precise narrative follows.

Energy is both wave and particle, light, and sound. It begins as silence and formless form, slowly changing in composition as its vibratory rates are reduced. A new understanding of light explains the journey of inorganic and organic matter from subtle energy to a frozen form of light–matter. This provides the foundations for the emerging new understanding of body, mind and spirit. We can start to know how we "fit" into the beautiful design of the cosmos.

Based on the continuing discoveries of science, contemporary physicians such as Gerber (2001) have envisioned a more comprehensive model for the human-energetic body (Figure 3.1).

His model depicts that the physical body is nested within a five-layer matrix of energy fields ranging from the well understood organic-molecular form of the physical body to organizational energies of higher energy sources. The total health of the human being is a product of a balanced and coordinated physical and higher dimensional homeostatic regulatory system (Gerber, 1995).

FIGURE 3.1

Human Bioenergetic System

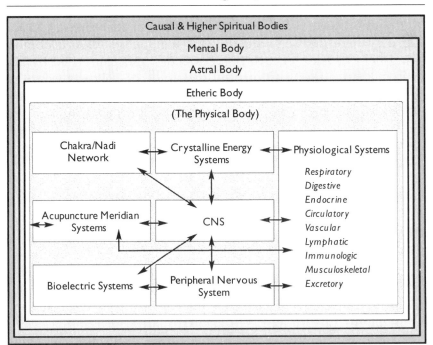

SOURCE: Adapted from R. Gerber (1995), *Vibrational medicine: New choices for healing ourselves* (Santa Fe, NM: Bear and Company), p. 420.

Tenet I on Human Bioenergetic System—Light

I-The physical body is a living photocell that is energized by the sun's light.

- Cell membrane is a liquid crystal semi-conductor with gates and channels that can be programmed like a computer chip.
- Cell membranes act like the cell's brain.
- Light stimulates the cell membrane's release of "protein gears" that initiate life sustaining processes.
- In living organisms, cells live in community.
- They share their awareness and coordinate their behaviors by releasing signal molecules into the environment.
- All cells commit to a common plan of action to assure the survival of the group/community.

Science of the Human Bioenergetic System

Since the beginning of time, humanity has utilized the energy and power of the sun. The human body is a living photocell that is energized by the sun's light. Nobel Prize winner Saent-Gyorgyi, recognized the impact of light and color on the human body, concluding that "all of the energy taken into our bodies is derived from the sun" (Szent-Gyorgyi, 1968). All human physiology including enzyme and hormonal systems involve the processing of light energy, causing dynamic reactions in the body. Light striking the body significantly alters basic biological cellular functioning and movement across cellular membranes. The energetic network, representing our physical/cellular framework, is organized and nourished by light.

At the cellular level, the wave patterns set in motion by light striking the body stimulate the Integral Membrane Proteins embedded in the cell membrane. The two classes of IMP complexes include *receptor proteins* and *effector proteins*. The receptor proteins act as "antenna" that read vibrational energy fields such as light, sound and wave frequencies. These proteins change shape and function, depending on the vibration striking the body, to carry its message into the cell. At this point the effector proteins engage in the appropriate life sustaining response. Thus the function of cells is derived from the movements of their "protein gears."

The interface between environmental signals and behavior-producing cytoplasmic proteins is the cell membrane which acts as the cell's brain. Crystals, structures with molecules arranged in regular and repetitive fashion, transmit energy waves through "vibratory messages" that guide cell function. Hard crystals are resilient minerals such as diamonds and rubies. Fluid crystals have molecules in a similar organized fashion, but arranged and bound together in a dynamic and easily adaptable manner. These crystals are found in digital watch faces and laptop computer screens. The cell membrane is a liquid crystal semiconductor with gates and channels, much like a computer chip. Both computers and cells are programmable, with the programmer outside of the computer/cell (Lipton, 2005, p. 90).

The protein complexes are the "perception switches" that stimulate the cell to respond in very basic ways to the potassium, calcium, oxygen, glucose, histamine, estrogen, toxins, light, or any number of other stimuli in their environment. When the cells respond, they release into the environment signals that influence the behavior of other cells within the ecosystem, creating a coordinated response. In living organisms, cells live in community where they share their "awareness" and coordinate their behaviors by releasing these "signal" molecules into the environment. All cells

---

Tenet II on Human Bioenergetic System—Beliefs

II-Beliefs influence and control biology.

- The same neural receptors that are found in the brain are present in most body cells.
- Perceptions, accurate or not, strongly impact our body-mind neural receptors.
- Molecules of emotion, generated by the brain, override the biological system, altering their built-in homeostatic mechanisms.
- Internal neurological structures relate to the expression of human consciousness:
  - Placebo Effect—the mind's positive suggestion can improve health
  - Nocebo Effect—a negative belief can deteriorate health.
- Over time our biological system adapts to our beliefs.

commit to a common plan of action that is coordinated by the brain, assuring survival of the host organism.

In her compelling work, *Molecules of Emotion*, Pert (1998) determined that the same "neural" receptors found in the brain were present on most of the body's cells. She demonstrated that the "mind" was not focused in the head but was distributed via signal molecules throughout the entire body. Along with feedback from the body's environmental information, "molecules of emotion" can be generated by the brain and override the biological system. A self-conscious mind can bring health or disease to the body if excessive stress is generated; beliefs control biology.

Our perceptions, whether accurate or not, strongly affect our body-mind. The well-known *placebo effect* has demonstrated that some people get well when they falsely believe they are getting medicine. Although it is known that the mind, through positive suggestion, improves health, it is also clear that unconstructive suggestions can damage health. These negative effects are referred to as the *nocebo effect*. Studies have shown that some patients who understood from their health care provider that they had a fatal diagnosis and "died of cancer" actually demonstrated—upon biopsy—to have very little disease present (Lipton, p. 142). By word and demeanor, physicians and other health care workers can convey hope-deflating messages to their patients. Positive and negative beliefs affect not only health but every aspect of life. Moreover, over time our biology adapts to those beliefs.

Emerging perspectives on the body–mind–spirit interconnection of humankind demonstrates more about the functioning of the human brain and how internal neurological structures relate to the expression of human consciousness. Simultaneously, scientific visionaries like Pribham (1998) are uncovering new relationships between chemistry, physics, and human brain physiology. Modeling through laser physics and holography demonstrates how a simple chemical reaction can contribute to the creation of a new order in neurological organization.

The holographic model of the universe gives a new foundation for comprehending the unseen energy interconnections between all things. At a microscopic level, we are all constructed from the same subatomic building blocks. At a macrocosmic level, we are each complex, yet uniquely arranged, aggregates of the same particularized energy field.

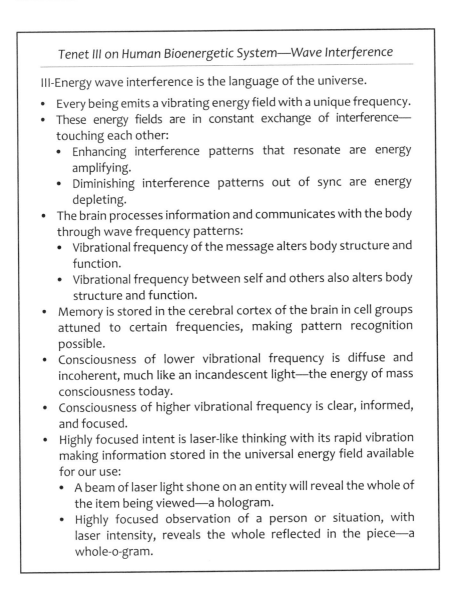

Tenet III on Human Bioenergetic System—Wave Interference

III-Energy wave interference is the language of the universe.

- Every being emits a vibrating energy field with a unique frequency.
- These energy fields are in constant exchange of interference—touching each other:
  - Enhancing interference patterns that resonate are energy amplifying.
  - Diminishing interference patterns out of sync are energy depleting.
- The brain processes information and communicates with the body through wave frequency patterns:
  - Vibrational frequency of the message alters body structure and function.
  - Vibrational frequency between self and others also alters body structure and function.
- Memory is stored in the cerebral cortex of the brain in cell groups attuned to certain frequencies, making pattern recognition possible.
- Consciousness of lower vibrational frequency is diffuse and incoherent, much like an incandescent light—the energy of mass consciousness today.
- Consciousness of higher vibrational frequency is clear, informed, and focused.
- Highly focused intent is laser-like thinking with its rapid vibration making information stored in the universal energy field available for our use:
  - A beam of laser light shone on an entity will reveal the whole of the item being viewed—a hologram.
  - Highly focused observation of a person or situation, with laser intensity, reveals the whole reflected in the piece—a whole-o-gram.

Wave interference is the language of the Universal Field. This pattern of interference is widely seen in nature. When two stones are dropped into a still pool of water, each creates a series of ever-expanding circular waves traveling outward. As the two groups of circular wave fronts meet, they interact and form an interference pattern. The pattern continues to expand, and at a specific point, the two merge into one larger, unified circle. Interference patterns can be enhancing (energy amplifying) when the waves are coordinated, as in harmonic resonance. Alternatively, the patterns can be diminishing (energy deflating), when the waves are out of sync.

Einstein's theory guides us into this unfolding world of energy through the use of laser light. Incandescent light from a light bulb is diffuse and incoherent, spreading a soft light over a large area. Laser light is a very special type of coherent light that is extremely orderly, with all waves moving in step, like soldiers marching. When light is highly focused, it can burn a hole through steel.

A hologram is made by sending a single laser beam through an optical beam splitter, creating two laser beams from the original one. When the pure, unaffected laser beam meets the reflected light from the second one, through a process of mirrors and plates, an interference pattern is created. This interference pattern is produced by the waves of one beam mixing and interacting with the waves of the other beam. The interference pattern created by laser light and captured on photographic film is what forms the hologram. When a pure beam of laser light is shone on any part of the photographic film, a three-dimensional view of the entire object is seen. Thus, a hologram is an energy interference pattern where each piece of the picture contains the whole.

Just as a laser light focused intensely on an object reveals the whole within one aspect observed, so too an authentic and unscripted observation about the person and/or situation in front of the nurse "now" will reveal the totality of the situation being cared for. This is the central physics precept behind "active observation," a witnessing function that transcends physical assessment.

The patterns of vibrational frequencies alter the physical and chemical properties of our brain, making new observations and memories possible. Talbot (1996) demonstrated that when we observe the world, the brain communicates with the rest of the body in the language of wave interference: the language of the spectrum domain—phase, amplitude, and frequency. In holographic fashion, the lens of the eye picks up certain interference patterns and converts them into three-dimensional images. We do not see the image on the back of our retina, but, rather, we create and project a virtual three-dimensional image of the object back into space, in the same place as the actual object.

In the act of "seeing," we transform the timeless, spaceless world of interference patterns into the concrete and discrete world of space and time. At this point, the image is collapsed and projected onto the retina, and our hand reaches out to touch the object where it really is, not inside our head.

Because our current reality is limited to recognizing information coming from the eye, we "see" only the observed, when in actuality we have the capacity to experience more fully a holographic view of the object. This holographic perspective encircles and penetrates the entirety of the field, giving us complete information, which, if we were open to recognizing, would tell us everything we need to know on an energetic/conscious level. It takes the initiation and opening of the third eye located in the brow chakra to recognize and understand this type of energy information.

As protons spin like magnets throughout the brain, they give off radiation. In this radiation is encoded wave information that can be used by the body to construct three-dimensional images of the body, the premise behind the MRI. Ongoing revolutionary research (Schempp, 1998) shows that this same principle is true for all biological systems. This unfolding work has led to the notion of "quantum holography."

Quantum fluctuations in the Universal Field hold infinite amounts of information, which can be recovered and reassembled into a three-dimensional image when perceived by a certain level of consciousness. The common consciousness of humankind is much like an incandescent light, diffuse and incoherent. When one focuses with a high degree of intent, such as during meditation, laser focus and an open mind make the information encoded in the Universal Energy Field available to us all. When we enter stillness, our attention shifts to the inner world of Spirit, which houses our soul and Spiritual Ego. From this vibrational level, we are connected to the Universal Field. And in that moment, all is revealed.

After seeing, the brain processes the information in the shorthand of wave frequency patterns and, like a local area network, dispenses this information throughout the brain in a highly distributed system of connections, where it is interpreted and stored. Storing the information in wave interference patterns is very efficient, allowing human memory to accommodate unimaginable quantities of data. It is estimated that with wave interference patterns, the entire U.S. Library of Congress book collection, virtually every book ever published in English, would fit onto a large sugar cube.

The patterns of vibrational frequencies alter our capacity for memory storage and retrieval as well (Mindell, 2004). Memory is distributed throughout the brain, with numerous cells of the cerebral cortex tuned into certain frequencies. Items of like frequency are stored together, making pattern recognition possible. The more often we see something "similar," the easier it is to recognize. It is this pattern recognition capacity—intuition—that marks the expert nurse. With one deep assessment, a number of possibilities are eliminated, while a select few probabilities emerge. It is an advantage to respond to a crisis from this "way of knowing." Simultaneously, when we habitually move in this direction, many subtle messages are missed that would add depth and richness to other possibilities when a situation is rich with complexity and does not demand an immediate response.

The brain also contains an "envelope," which limits the amount of wave information available to it as a protection against the limitless wave information contained in the Universal Field. When we are encouraged to "push the envelope," it is a metaphor for enlarging the consciousness or wave capacity of the brain. Exercising our capacity for a shift in focus from analysis to attention enlarges the size of the envelope.

Tenet IV on Human Bioenergetic System—Epigenetics

IV-Epigenetics has identified mechanisms that transcend and override DNA coding.

- Every cell contains the master DNA blueprint with enough information to create an entire human body.
- A vital etheric field of energy information wraps around the physical body, providing the blueprint for its development and maintenance.
- DNA blueprints passed on through the genes are not set in concrete and can be overridden by the vibrational interference of strong emotions.
- Illness is more commonly caused by environmentally induced (nutrition, stress, emotions) epigenetic alterations than defective genes from heredity.

This model increases our understanding of the bioenergetic fields associated with the physical-chemical structure of the human body and the cell. The holographic principle that "every piece contains the whole" is also seen in the cellular structure of all living beings. Every cell contains the master DNA blueprint with enough information to create an entire human body, instructing each cell how to grow and function. This principle underlies the cloning of living cells (Gerber, 2001).

Epigenetics has uncovered a complex three-dimensional map of a bioenergetic field that surrounds the physical body. This field, or "vital body," wraps around the physical body, carrying coded information for the spatial organization of the human body as well as a roadmap for cellular repair (Pray, 2004; Silverman, 2004). It also is the primary "energy source" for the body, giving us the vitality needed for daily life.

DNA blueprints passed on through genes are not set in concrete. Environmental influences such as nutrition, stress, and emotions can modify these genes, significantly altering their manifestation. In their compelling book on The Lamarckian Dimension, Jablonka and Lamb observed (Jablonka & Lamb, 1995, p. 178):

> In recent years, molecular biology has shown that the genome is far more fluid and responsive to the environment than previously supposed. It has also shown that information can be transmitted to descendants in ways other than through the base sequence of DNA.

Multiple studies have demonstrated epigenetic mechanisms as a significant factor in a variety of diseases such as cancer and heart disease. One study showed that only 5% of cancer and cardiovascular patients can attribute their disorder to heredity (Willett, 2002). Malignancies are derived primarily from environmentally induced epigenetic alterations and not defective genes (Baylin, 1997; Jones, 2001; Kling, 2003; Seppa, 2000). The evidence increasingly shows a deep connection between an organism and its emotional environment. Vital well-being requires a dynamic balance between the physical body and its higher dimensional homeostatic regulatory system.

THE HUMAN MIND RE-VISIONED—
AN EXPANSIVE FIELD OF CONSCIOUSNESS

Simply everything, living and inorganic, is shaped from the same matter that exists throughout the physical universe—energy. Somehow, consciousness participates in this entire process. We experience the outer physical world as external to us, while we also experience an inner world of awareness called Soul Consciousness. Consciousness itself is a form of energy, and at the highest levels it integrates all life processes. It is coextensive in the universe and exists in all matter. Each individual and human-kind as a species are identified by their patterns of consciousness. A person does not *possess* consciousness, the person *is* conscious-ness. Consciousness (awareness) is the ground of all being, the ground of both mind and matter (Laszlo & Currivan, 2008).

The new model for the contemporary human being includes consciousness at various stages of manifestation from the visible outer world of manifest thought to the subjective inner world of abstract thought and the middle mental-reflective world of mind that unites them. These three worlds are wrapped in the Causal Body, a world of higher energy serving as the outer sheath of our bioenergetic body. It is the home of our Soul.

Our personal stage of development is manifest in terms of behaviors that reflect our "inner" and "outer" worldview, our per-ceptual capacity within those spheres. Continuing spiritual devel-opment of the soul occurs as we increasingly incorporate higher levels of awareness into our basic way of being in the objective world of form (Fisher, 1996b, pp. 58–62).

Science of Consciousness

Consciousness is the informational capacity of a system, the degree of its capacity to interact with its environment (Chopra, 2009). It is demonstrated by the degree of autonomy a system gains in dynamic relationship with its environment. Even the simplest one-cell organisms have a primitive form of consciousness. As the quality of consciousness increases so does vibrational frequency. The number and variety of responses to the environment also expand. This is manifest as a movement from reaction to a greater repertoire of responses with ease, speed, and grace, the result of greater refinement of perception in terms of insight, context, and detail.

The vibrational capacity of each level of being is not the same. Our reality depends on where we are on the spectrum of consciousness: level of consciousness determines reality. The consciousness of human awareness encompasses plant and animal ranges as well as astral and spiritual realms. Increasing awareness creates a more intricate nervous system capable of environmental interaction in a more complex pattern (Figure 3.2).

Viewing matter as a manifestation of consciousness reaffirms the unitary nature of body-mind, with mind representing faster high-frequency energy waves and body, slower and lower amplitude. "Absolute Consciousness is a state in which contrasting

FIGURE 3.2

Vibrational Fields and Consciousness

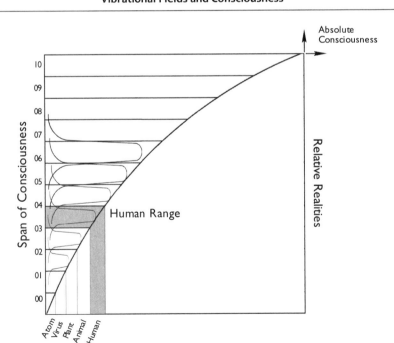

SOURCE: Adapted from I. Bentov (1978), *Stalking the wild pendulum* (New York: E. P. Dutton), p. 80.

Tenet I on Spheres of Consciousness—Outer World

I-The Objective Universe—Essence of Outer World

Function: Low vibration level that allows consciousness to express itself in concrete life forms and life experiences.

- Experienced as the body, personality, ego, and Lower mind (central nervous system [CNS]/Brain)
- Outer manifestation of our level of consciousness
- Is the vehicle that allows us to experience life.

---

concepts become reconciled and fused. Movement and rest fuse into one at the Source" (Bentov, 1978).

The new model for human-energy physiology includes consciousness at various stages of expression in each human being. Just as the bioenergetic body is composed of five specific "levels of energy," individual perception is uniquely different within each of these Spheres of Consciousness.

The outer world is composed of all things material. It is the world of experience in all its infinite beauty and challenge. One of the many forms of life on the planet, the human species alone has a capacity for conscious awareness greater and more innovative than that of others. The human body impacts and is impacted by the constant interactive dance of energy in the environment. Others experience us as this physical body with specific characteristics and an ego personality style that is a rich blend of our beliefs, expectations, and attitudes about simply everything. This rich mixture of elements is our unique thumbprint on the world.

The intermediate mental-reflective sphere is the middle ground of our existence—the place our conscious awareness resides. Germinal thought forms that are generated in our higher subjective mind are brought into material manifestation through this portal. As abstract thought enters this realm, the vibration is slowed down and focused by our intent into a certain form of manifestation. The body-mind will take the information and translate it into concrete form within the body or physical action of the body. It is also the doorway for the Soul to contact and influence the personality. The more our focus turns inward, the greater is the engagement of the Soul.

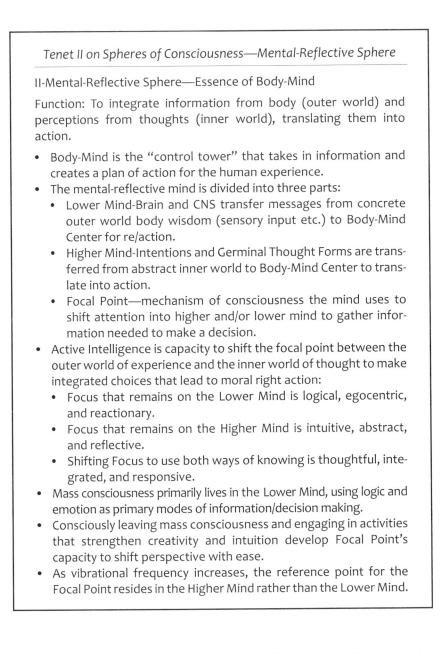

Tenet II on Spheres of Consciousness—Mental-Reflective Sphere

II-Mental-Reflective Sphere—Essence of Body-Mind

Function: To integrate information from body (outer world) and perceptions from thoughts (inner world), translating them into action.

- Body-Mind is the "control tower" that takes in information and creates a plan of action for the human experience.
- The mental-reflective mind is divided into three parts:
  - Lower Mind-Brain and CNS transfer messages from concrete outer world body wisdom (sensory input etc.) to Body-Mind Center for re/action.
  - Higher Mind-Intentions and Germinal Thought Forms are transferred from abstract inner world to Body-Mind Center to translate into action.
  - Focal Point—mechanism of consciousness the mind uses to shift attention into higher and/or lower mind to gather information needed to make a decision.
- Active Intelligence is capacity to shift the focal point between the outer world of experience and the inner world of thought to make integrated choices that lead to moral right action:
  - Focus that remains on the Lower Mind is logical, egocentric, and reactionary.
  - Focus that remains on the Higher Mind is intuitive, abstract, and reflective.
  - Shifting Focus to use both ways of knowing is thoughtful, integrated, and responsive.
- Mass consciousness primarily lives in the Lower Mind, using logic and emotion as primary modes of information/decision making.
- Consciously leaving mass consciousness and engaging in activities that strengthen creativity and intuition develop Focal Point's capacity to shift perspective with ease.
- As vibrational frequency increases, the reference point for the Focal Point resides in the Higher Mind rather than the Lower Mind.

The abstract, creative, and spiritual dimension of being is the inner subjective dimension of consciousness. Energy is vibrating so rapidly that it is experienced as images, concepts, or germinal thought forms rather than words. It is the dwelling place of our

---

Tenet III on Spheres of Consciousness—Inner World

III-Subjective Universe—Essence of Inner World

Function: The internal world of beliefs, intentions, creativity, and wisdom that informs and forms Outer World experience.

- Vibration is so rapid that it cannot be molded into thought forms.
- Abstract thought field germinates intangible ideas and broad concepts.
- Focused intention creates outcomes imagined by slowing down vibration toward a specific goal.
- Slower vibration enters mind to be combined with logic as decision is made.
- Intuition recognizes repeating life lessons encoded as patterns of information stored in the brain.
- When something is observed as "off-pattern," an intuitive flash occurs before it becomes manifest in the outer world.
- Intuitive nurses "sense" something is wrong and intervene before the problem becomes evident.

Spiritual Ego, which coordinates our intent with deep wisdom and love, a higher consciousness focused on higher good. This inner wisdom balances to ego personality, which often makes decisions based on best interests of the self.

After building a strong foundation in the outer world, we increasingly focus on inner development. As our vibratory pattern increases, we move more easily in this realm, becoming perceptive, creative, intuitive, joyful, and morally guided.

The soul holds the seed crystal of our destiny and life purpose, our authentic self. Our unique potential and our conscience reside here. Universal spiritual qualities possessed by all, such as love, joy, and gratitude, can also be connected through this space. It is here that our healing presence resides and connects with the heart space of others. When our vibrational capacity is high enough, our upper mind engages with intuition—and wisdom is awakened along with universal qualities of the Spirit, which reside in the Causal Body (next Tenet). This deeper consciousness transcends the limitations of thought, infusing our life with synchronicities as we live the path of our divine destiny.

Tenet IV on Spheres of Consciousness—The Soul

IV-The Soul—Essence of Being

Function: Unique dimension of each individual holding their destiny blueprint.

- Home of the authenticity of each person
- Anchored in a sixth-dimensional space vortex outside the heart chakra (it is unseen by humans who can perceive only four-dimensional forms)
- Serves as the unifying force integrating human consciousness between its concrete, physical, and abstract spiritual experiences in this lifetime
- When our vibrational capacity is sufficiently high, it resonates with this coalescing force field and Intuition—our Inner Wisdom—is awakened.

Tenet V on Spheres of Consciousness—Causal Body

V-The Causal Body—Vehicle of Consciousness

Function: Outer sheath protecting our entire bioenergetic body vibrating so rapidly it is experienced as silence.

- Shaped like a luminous egg, it encases the entire energy field of the person
- Repository of the essence of all our previous life experiences and the Spark of Life that infuses the Soul with Spirit
- Contains Universal Wisdom and Spiritual Qualities, such as love, peace, and compassion
- Interface through which our energetic vibratory patterns interact with the energy matrix of the Universe in a specific wave interference pattern that is our identity signature in the cosmos.

Spirit interacts with, and manifests through, the many forms of physical matter. The journey of spirit through the worlds of matter provides the strongest driving force for the evolutionary process. We touch this level of Consciousness only when in deep states of meditation and silence. A moment in this space can change perception forever. Unsustainable, we touch this space, only to return with more love and compassion to share with the world.

> It is the enriching endowing power of spirit that moves, inspires and breathes life into that vehicle we perceive as the physical body. A system of medicine which denies or ignores its existence will be incomplete, because it leaves out the most fundamental quality of human existence—the spiritual dimension (Gerber, p. 419).

Our personal level of consciousness is described in terms that relate to our "inner" and "outer" perceptional capacity within those spheres. Continuing spiritual development of the soul occurs as we increase the incorporation of higher levels of awareness into our basic human condition in the objective world of form (Fisher, 1996b, pp. 58–62).

SCIENCE OF ENERGY FIELDS

Most current notions, stemming from Newton's mechanical view, believe that the human body is a complex machine. Expanding our worldview toward Einstein's physics perspective, we see the human being as a multidimensional organism, composed of physical cellular systems in dynamic exchange with complex and diverse regulatory energetic fields. In this vibrant and dynamic world, health includes the subtle-energy fields surrounding the body along with the cells and organs that comprise it. The belief that we are frail biochemical machines controlled by genes is being usurped by the knowledge that we are the powerful and conscious creators of our lives and the world in which we live.

Realities of spirit do not negate laws of science; they only extend them to include higher frequency dimensions, much as the incorporation of quantum principles into mechanical science increased the understanding and integration of various laws and principles that appeared disconnected in a three-dimensional world.

The creative potential embedded within Absolute Consciousness (the Universal Zero-Point Field) has a self-organizing capacity that influences the being who perceives it.

The force of life continuously moves toward higher order, from planetary motion to the functioning of society. Prigogine's Theory of Dissipative Structures (1976) demonstrates that while all dynamic systems fluctuate, rather than evening out, they eventually move to some supraordinate shift. The new order appears when a giant fluctuation is stabilized through an exchange of amplified energy with its environment. The functional and stable element is impacted by chance factors or critical events, coupled with an energetic surge, which results in a shift that produces physical mutations or behavioral or biological change.

Sheldrake (1981), a cellular biologist, demonstrated the mechanism for a shift in capacity for an individual as well as a species. His research showed that characteristic forms and behavior of physical, chemical, and biological systems are determined by invisible organizing fields acting across time and space. These morphogenetic fields are without mass or energy and are cumulative in nature. Each generation can acquire learned tasks more easily than the last because of capacity embedded within this field. At some critical juncture, the acquired function is transcended into higher order and form because a morphogenetic field has been enlarged; this is the evolutionary nature of life.

These new models give us a view of the human body as a complex system composed of both matter and energy that are intertwined at multiple levels of reality. The image of the body as five nested hierarchies was discovered in India as part of the Vedanta literature. It also appears in Judaic tradition as part of the Kabala as well as in the ancient mystery schools of Egypt (Bly, 1977; Frawley, 1989; Svoboda & Lade, 1995).

How this translates into body–mind–spirit connection is one of the most beautiful discoveries of modern day science. The five "bodies" comprise the human condition, and the way they dance together is poetry in motion, a true work of art.

The Gross Physical Body is the coarsest level, an inert mineral machine, penetrated atom for atom by the vital body. It is the most organized and highly evolved as well as the most highly crystallized of all forms of matter in the Universe. Each human body, the medium through which Consciousness experiences life, is unique because of its physical structure. It serves as the receptor and transmitter through which are expressed the vital, emotional, and mental vibrations/messages that originate in the subtle bodies

---

Tenet I of Energy Anatomy—Gross Physical Body

I-Gross Physical Body:

Primary Function: To provide a functioning vehicle to engage with life in the material world.

- The Gross Physical Body is an inert mineral machine, penetrated atom for atom by the vital body (next tenet).
- It is the most organized and highly evolved and the most highly crystallized of all forms of matter in the universe.
- Each body is unique because of its physical structure.
- Body intelligence is oriented to physical sensation: sight, sound, smell, taste, touch, the immunosystem, and the hormonal system (flight/fight response).
- Subtle-energy bodies surround, inform, and vitalize it (vital, emotional, mental, causal).
- It serves as the receptor and transmitter to express the vital, emotional, and mental vibrations/messages that originate in the subtle bodies.
- It is the medium through which consciousness experiences life.
- It can be further developed through proper nutrition, rest, and exercise.

Illness:

- Disease occurs when normal body chemistry or physics goes awry.
- Chronic illness occurs when emotional/belief systems go awry.
- Injury occurs when body is impacted by external agents such as microbes or trauma.
- Allopathic medical practices such as surgery, drugs, and radiation are appropriate treatments, especially when fast results are desired.

---

that surround and inform it. The physical body is not a fixed entity. It can be further developed through proper nutrition, rest, and exercise.

The physical level of disease is well known to the world of Western medicine. Illness occurs when the body's normal chemistry or physics goes awry. It also can be impacted by external agents such as microbes or trauma. Allopathic medicine, like classic physics, is very appropriate in treating mechanical and traumatic injuries, especially when immediate results are needed. Conventional medicine with its practices of surgery, drugs, and radiation assists with control or removal of physical symptoms.

Tenet II of Energy Anatomy—Vital Body

II-Vital Body:

Primary Function: This three-dimensional body vitalizes and energizes the dense physical body, functioning as an intermediary for transmission of force-matter (coalescing energy that is slowing into form) radiating from the emotional and mental bodies to the physical brain and nervous system.

- It is an exact copy of the physical body.
- It permeates through and follows the contours of the body while extending 3 to 5 centimeters beyond it.
- It is composed of colorless, volatile liquid ether.
- Its primary vortex for entry into the body is located by the spleen chakra.
- This energy wrapper provides the structural and functional blueprints for the forms and programs of various organic structures.
- It guides the process of differentiation of a single-celled embryo into a biological body of discriminate organs.
- The blueprints guide vital body functions as well as maintenance, reproduction, and so on.
- It removes and cleanses the physical body of depleted etheric atoms much as the circulatory system nourishes and cleanses the physical body.
- The vital body is often referred to as "the aura."
- Morphogenesis can also influence the vital body through access to nonphysical and nonlocal energy fields.

Illness:

- Physical disease is a manifestation of disrupted vital life force, resulting in imbalances between physical and vital bodies.
- Illness results in symptoms of blocked energy between the physical and vital body, that is, congestion, aching, and tightness around the body.
- Physical symptoms also accompany recognizable symptoms of distressed body organs when they become depleted/affected.
- Homeopathy, Eastern Ayurveda, and Chinese Medicine focus on restoring the blueprints of the vital body.
- Blueprint restoration is a lengthy process, so often Allopathic and Homeopathic remedies are given simultaneously.

The Vital Body serves two purposes: it provides vital energy to the dense physical body, and it functions as an intermediate for the transmission of force matter (coalescing energy that is turning into form) from the vibrational emissions of the emotional and mental bodies to the physical brain and nervous system. (Fisher, 1996a, pp. 2–4, 29–34; Mindell, 2004).

Current discussions in the scientific world are exploring the electromagnetic and gravitational force field of energy through the "String Theory" paradigm (Green, 1999). It states that each quanta of energy is, in the final analysis, not a point but rather a tiny, vibrating, one-dimensional loop similar to a very thin rubber band. Everything at the microscopic level consists of combinations of vibrating strands whose mass and force changes are determined by its vibratory pattern. Spirillae are the fundamental energy forms through which various levels of energy (consciousness) are manifest throughout the Universe (Figure 3.3).

FIGURE 3.3

Energy Spirillae

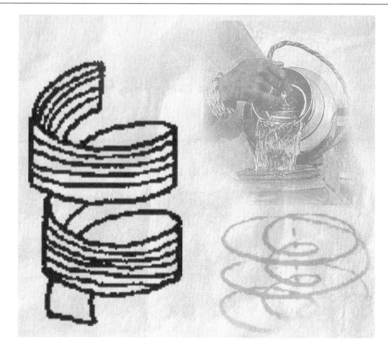

SOURCE: Adapted from B.S. Fisher (1996a), *Man, grand reflection of greater cosmos: Studies in occult anatomy* (Vol.3) (Prescott, AZ: Subru Publications), p. 21.

Emerging as a Vital Life Force from the sun, energy spirillae are converted into "Vitality Globules" as energy and nourishment for the body (Fisher, pp. 23–25). These Globules, etheric corpuscles, are absorbed by the vital body through force center openings (chakras) located just outside the physical body. The largest vortex is located near the spleen chakra. Just as a prism refracts light waves into seven colors representing the differing vibratory levels of light energy, the spleen refracts particles (frozen light) into seven color globules of Vital Life Force, which nourish the seven chakra centers along with the specific endocrine glands and nerve structures they support. Simultaneously, excess Vital Force and depleted etheric "atoms," some chemical molecules, and microorganisms are eliminated through the vital aura, detoxifying the physical body, much as the circulatory system supports the physical body. Conservation and appropriate use of our Vital Force are essential to physical and extrasensory (emotional-mental) health (Figure 3.4).

FIGURE 3.4

Vitality Globules

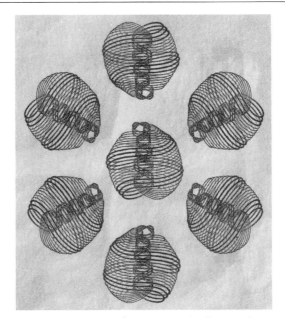

SOURCE: Adapted from B.S. Fisher (1996), *Man, grand reflection of greater cosmos: Studies in occult anatomy* (Vol. 3) (Prescott, AZ: Subru Publications), p. 25.

The vital body's second and higher function is the transmission of emotional/mental force-matter. It organizes and separates the "higher" ethers, concerned with sense perception and memory, from the "lower" ethers involved with vitalizing, maintaining, and propagating the dense physical body. The lower part remains with the dense body to keep it alive, whereas the higher part is used by the ego as an organ of sense perception, serving as the foundation of the body-mind. It can be strengthened through repetition of aesthetic and altruistic practices.

Each vital body is unique because of conditioning. Certain blueprints are used more than others, creating a pattern of personality. This "etheric double" serves as a medium for the Life Force, which affects vitality, assimilation and growth, excretion and detoxification, sense perception, and memory of immediate life events, our *body-mind* impressions.

Disease is a manifestation of disrupted body plans in the morphogenetic field resulting in imbalances between physical and vital bodies. As this is the body sensation level of consciousness, illness elicits certain feelings or symptoms that accompany the recognizable physical components. Homeopathy as well as Eastern Ayurveda and Chinese Medicine are focused on treating the vital body. Restoring the blueprints takes more time than addressing physical symptoms. Often a blending of conventional and holistic care in a compatible fashion begins to foster healing at deeper levels of being.

The Desire/Emotional Body resides in a world that is primarily one of color; a four-dimensional world where time, space, motion, and gravitational laws differ from the physical world. Sensitive to color vibrations, vision is four dimensional, with objects being viewed from all sides simultaneously. The rapid circulation within the field precludes formation of localized centers of perception; emotions are "free floating" feelings as they are sensed all along the outer edge of the ovoid border of the emotional body. Here subtle attraction and repulsion, interest and disinterest are born.

Thoughts and emotions impact the vital body primarily through the CNS and the crown chakra. In an emotionally healthy person, the flow of particle-wave exchange is effortless and light. However, a burst of negative emotions or aggression forms a clotting of this energy causing stagnation from loss of flow, much as a

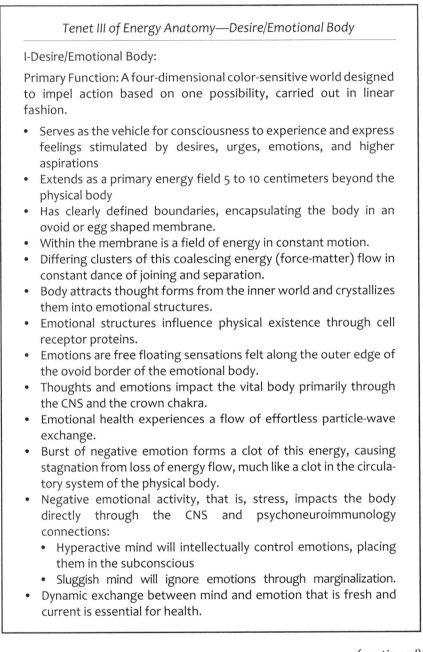

Tenet III of Energy Anatomy—Desire/Emotional Body

I-Desire/Emotional Body:

Primary Function: A four-dimensional color-sensitive world designed to impel action based on one possibility, carried out in linear fashion.

- Serves as the vehicle for consciousness to experience and express feelings stimulated by desires, urges, emotions, and higher aspirations
- Extends as a primary energy field 5 to 10 centimeters beyond the physical body
- Has clearly defined boundaries, encapsulating the body in an ovoid or egg shaped membrane.
- Within the membrane is a field of energy in constant motion.
- Differing clusters of this coalescing energy (force-matter) flow in constant dance of joining and separation.
- Body attracts thought forms from the inner world and crystallizes them into emotional structures.
- Emotional structures influence physical existence through cell receptor proteins.
- Emotions are free floating sensations felt along the outer edge of the ovoid border of the emotional body.
- Thoughts and emotions impact the vital body primarily through the CNS and the crown chakra.
- Emotional health experiences a flow of effortless particle-wave exchange.
- Burst of negative emotion forms a clot of this energy, causing stagnation from loss of energy flow, much like a clot in the circulatory system of the physical body.
- Negative emotional activity, that is, stress, impacts the body directly through the CNS and psychoneuroimmunology connections:
  - Hyperactive mind will intellectually control emotions, placing them in the subconscious
  - Sluggish mind will ignore emotions through marginalization.
- Dynamic exchange between mind and emotion that is fresh and current is essential for health.

(continued)

Tenet III of Energy Anatomy—Desire/Emotional Body (continued)

Illness:

- Disease is manifest as depression, anxiety, anger, fear, or apathy due to energy stagnation or loss of energy flow from clotting.
- Balance between mind-body must be restored for healing to occur.
- Healing methods include biofeedback, meditation, yoga, and color therapy.
- If disease entity also includes the mental body, as in mental illness, this form of intervention is inadequate.

---

stroke in the vascular system of the physical body. Negative mental activity affects the body directly through the brain's connection to the CNS as well as through newly discovered psychoneuroimmunology neuropeptide connections.

The mind reacts to stress-producing agents, determining whether their effects will have an adverse reaction to the vital and physical body. An individual develops conditioned responses over time, ascribing meaning to the event with a patterned mental quality. The hyperactive mind will intellectualize and control emotions, burying the issue in the subconscious, whereas the sluggish mind will ignore the event, placing it into the realm of the subconscious through marginalization. A healthy balance of mind and emotion that transcends conditioning in a creative and fresh way is essential for healing at this level. Restoring balance at this level involves mind-body healing methods such as meditation, biofeedback, and yoga.

The Mental Reflective Body is preeminently a vibrational frequency of tone; good music inspires us. We can "hear" what is being said, but we know the truth of it by what is "felt" behind the word. This is our Thought World, the *true home of the human mind*. It is a five-dimensional world, the added dimension being consciousness of more than one possibility within an event. It allows us to make choices that are more intelligent from the "clear head" in a difficult situation versus the perspective of more-limited four-dimensional consciousness in which only one possibility at a time can be seen in linear fashion.

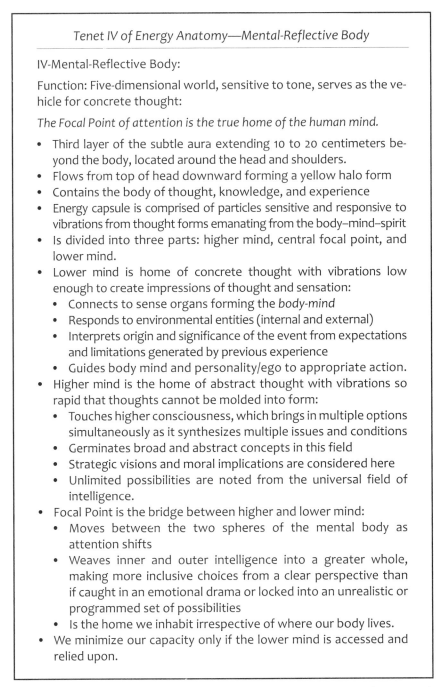

Tenet IV of Energy Anatomy—Mental-Reflective Body

IV-Mental-Reflective Body:

Function: Five-dimensional world, sensitive to tone, serves as the vehicle for concrete thought:

The Focal Point of attention is the true home of the human mind.

- Third layer of the subtle aura extending 10 to 20 centimeters beyond the body, located around the head and shoulders.
- Flows from top of head downward forming a yellow halo form
- Contains the body of thought, knowledge, and experience
- Energy capsule is comprised of particles sensitive and responsive to vibrations from thought forms emanating from the body–mind–spirit
- Is divided into three parts: higher mind, central focal point, and lower mind.
- Lower mind is home of concrete thought with vibrations low enough to create impressions of thought and sensation:
  - Connects to sense organs forming the *body-mind*
  - Responds to environmental entities (internal and external)
  - Interprets origin and significance of the event from expectations and limitations generated by previous experience
  - Guides body mind and personality/ego to appropriate action.
- Higher mind is the home of abstract thought with vibrations so rapid that thoughts cannot be molded into form:
  - Touches higher consciousness, which brings in multiple options simultaneously as it synthesizes multiple issues and conditions
  - Germinates broad and abstract concepts in this field
  - Strategic visions and moral implications are considered here
  - Unlimited possibilities are noted from the universal field of intelligence.
- Focal Point is the bridge between higher and lower mind:
  - Moves between the two spheres of the mental body as attention shifts
  - Weaves inner and outer intelligence into a greater whole, making more inclusive choices from a clear perspective than if caught in an emotional drama or locked into an unrealistic or programmed set of possibilities
  - Is the home we inhabit irrespective of where our body lives.
- We minimize our capacity only if the lower mind is accessed and relied upon.

(continued)

Tenet IV of Energy Anatomy—Mental-Reflective Body (continued)

Illness:

- Disease is manifest by chronic confusion or indecision, dogmatic beliefs, programmed thoughts/responses, irrational thought patterns, and inflexible rigidity.
- Easier to modify or purify quickly due to low degree of organization or crystallization unless it involves significant mental illness.
- Therapies include activities that strengthen abstract thought and intuition and aesthetic practices, such as art or music appreciation that strengthen recognition of symbols and metaphors.

Mind is the connecting point between the lower realm of "analytic thought" and the higher realm of "abstract thought." It is here, in the organized and specialized body of the Thought World, that a bridge connects the lower bodies (which comprise the personality ego) with the higher bodies (Spiritual Ego) (Figure 3.5).

The lower aspect of our mental body connects with our sense organs, forming the *body-mind,* which responds to environmental entities (internal and external) that act on the body. We embody "seven senses"; sight, touch, hearing, smell, taste, the immunosystem, and the endocrine system. Body awareness notifies the brain (physical brain or cell receptors) that something is in the environment. Externally, we react (move hand from hot stove); while, physiologically, a toxic invader alerts the immunosystem or a stressful event compels the endocrine system to prepare the body for quick response. The concrete mind interprets the origin and significance of the event, deciding if the issue is threatening or enabling, guiding the body-mind in an appropriate reaction.

The higher aspect of our mental body is accessed through aesthetic or abstract thoughts, performing its most important function as the gateway through which the Spiritual Ego contacts, controls, and "dwells within" the lower vehicles that form the personality. It is the doorway to Intuition and our Higher Wisdom.

The Causal Body, theosophical term, is viewed as the outer sheath or Vehicle of Consciousness of the Spirit. It holds our

FIGURE 3.5

Mental Reflective Body

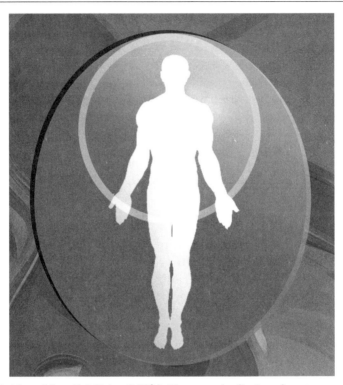

SOURCE: Adapted from B.S. Fisher (1996a), *Man, grand reflection of greater cosmos: Studies in occult anatomy* (Vol.3) (Prescott, AZ: Subru Publications), p. 15.

universal archetype, built through successive incarnations, forming our unique inner identity. It has a very resilient outer "skin" of protective film that serves as a protection against external forces and influences, while also providing the connection point to the Universal Energy Field, the Source. Every thought, feeling and experience we have influences All-That-Is vibrationally. We are One.

The Causal Body is a six-dimensional world with the addition of transcendent consciousness, which facilitates identifying all possibilities existing at once. Vibration is of the highest rate in consciousness and is experienced when touched into as silence or stillness. This "highest" form of expression is our immortal one, the seat of our individuality that persists from life to life, the vehicle of consciousness of the reincarnating Soul.

Tenet V of Energy Anatomy—Causal Body

V-Causal Body:

Primary Function: This six-dimensional world is our vehicle of consciousness that houses our Spirit—Spark of Life, identifying all possibilities in multidimensional space simultaneously.

- Vibration is so rapid that it is experienced as silence.
- Blue oval extending 50 to 60 centimeters beyond the physical body, serving as an outer sheath to the other four bodies of consciousness
- Resilient and elastic outer skin, which allows it to flex and change without breaking
- Serves as protection against external forces and influences
- Provides connection point to the Universal Energy Field, the Source
- Holds the archetypes of humanity and forms our inner identity
- Home of universal spiritual qualities, such as peace and compassion, found equally in the entire human race.
- Spirit facilitates the highest form of self-expression, our immortal individuality that persists from one lifetime to another as the vehicle of consciousness for our reincarnating soul
- Soul is the blueprint for this incarnation and serves as the repository of all knowledge, faculties, and spiritually worthwhile experiences accumulated in this lifetime.
- Intuition—inner wisdom—opens access for our reflective mind to our soul's knowledge repository and influence, which directs us on our path of destiny.
- Soul has access to the Causal Body, and when the vibrational frequency is sufficiently rapid, the Universal Spiritual Qualities can also be accessed and incorporated.
- Distillation of the essence of all bodily experiences provides energetic nourishment for transformation of our spiritual nature.
- Unity-wholeness is experienced when our authentic life (soul destiny) is guided by our Spiritual Ego, and our "essence" vibrates at the level of universal spiritual qualities, connecting us to all.

Illness:

- Disease is lack of conscious awareness or connection to our Higher Self, which results in a restless melancholy or longing.

(continued)

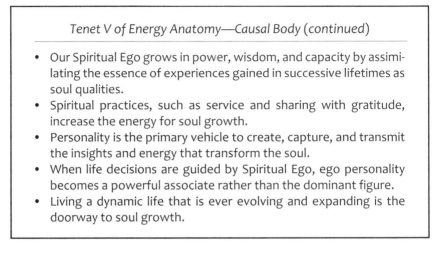

Tenet V of Energy Anatomy—Causal Body (continued)

- Our Spiritual Ego grows in power, wisdom, and capacity by assimilating the essence of experiences gained in successive lifetimes as soul qualities.
- Spiritual practices, such as service and sharing with gratitude, increase the energy for soul growth.
- Personality is the primary vehicle to create, capture, and transmit the insights and energy that transform the soul.
- When life decisions are guided by Spiritual Ego, ego personality becomes a powerful associate rather than the dominant figure.
- Living a dynamic life that is ever evolving and expanding is the doorway to soul growth.

The Causal Body also holds the Universal Spiritual Qualities found in every human being; love, compassion, peace, gratitude, and so on. In moments of meditation or enlightenment, we can touch into this space and acquire these qualities into our Soul. Others will recognize them in us, even if they do not yet have a direct connection to their own capacities. This fosters a sense of trust and oneness, an important element in Healing Presence.

The Soul is the mediator between the Mental-Reflective Body and the Causal Body. Tapping into our intuition, referred to as "Inner Wisdom," gives us access to the soul's repository of all knowledge, faculties, and spiritually worthwhile experiences accumulated during many lifetimes as well as the seed crystal for this lifetime. Spiritual practices assist the Soul in vibrating to the level of the Causal Body to acquire insights and instructions from the Universal Field.

THE HUMAN BEING REVISITED— DYNAMIC BODY–MIND–SPIRIT BALANCE

Although contemporary nurses are expert at ways of knowing and monitoring the homeostatic mechanisms of the physical body, we know less about the more subtle bodies that surround and support it. How does energy move into the concrete body to stimulate the multiple coordinating activities that support its function? And

---

Basic Tenets of the Chakra System

I The Root Chakra:

Function: Creates the necessary foundation for life and living

Consciousness Level: Animalistic level

- Activated at birth when the umbilical cord is cut
- Vital energy channeled into this chakra creates a deep connection with the world
- Energizes the physical body, lower extremities, including the feet.
- Establishes and maintains physical connection with the world
- Located at the base of the tailbone (red) and connected to the sacral-coccygeal nerve plexus
- Energizes suprarenal glands; cortisone, adrenalin, noradrenalin.

II The Sacral Chakra

Function: Activates all senses

Consciousness Level: Mass consciousness level

- Provides sexual and creative energy as well as instinctual and emotional feelings
- Boosts our awareness of and desire for beauty, relationships, and pleasure
- Establishes a healthy enthusiasm for being alive
- Expresses the EROS aspect of love
- Located in the lower abdomen (orange) near the spleen, bladder, and lower intestines as well as sacral nerve plexus
- Energizes testicles and ovaries; estrogen and testosterone.

III Solar Plexus Chakra:

Function: Serves as gateway for emotions and the projection of volitional energy (such as anger)

Consciousness Level: Aspiration level

- Intellectually, it determines our level of decision making, direction, and personal power
- Emotionally, it guides our ability to trust our most fundamental intuition and instincts
- Sustains our self-image and personality formed by the masks, characters, and attitudes we adopt to navigate through the world.
- Provides the determination, conviction, and courage to achieve the life we are seeking

---

(continued)

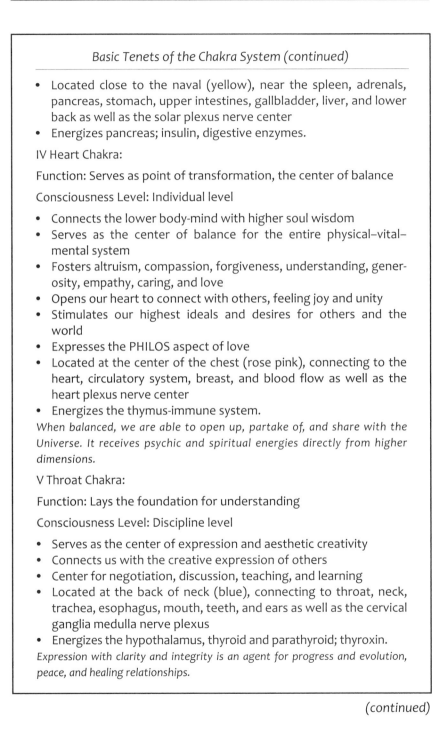

Basic Tenets of the Chakra System (continued)

- Located close to the naval (yellow), near the spleen, adrenals, pancreas, stomach, upper intestines, gallbladder, liver, and lower back as well as the solar plexus nerve center
- Energizes pancreas; insulin, digestive enzymes.

IV Heart Chakra:

Function: Serves as point of transformation, the center of balance

Consciousness Level: Individual level

- Connects the lower body-mind with higher soul wisdom
- Serves as the center of balance for the entire physical–vital–mental system
- Fosters altruism, compassion, forgiveness, understanding, generosity, empathy, caring, and love
- Opens our heart to connect with others, feeling joy and unity
- Stimulates our highest ideals and desires for others and the world
- Expresses the PHILOS aspect of love
- Located at the center of the chest (rose pink), connecting to the heart, circulatory system, breast, and blood flow as well as the heart plexus nerve center
- Energizes the thymus-immune system.

When balanced, we are able to open up, partake of, and share with the Universe. It receives psychic and spiritual energies directly from higher dimensions.

V Throat Chakra:

Function: Lays the foundation for understanding

Consciousness Level: Discipline level

- Serves as the center of expression and aesthetic creativity
- Connects us with the creative expression of others
- Center for negotiation, discussion, teaching, and learning
- Located at the back of neck (blue), connecting to throat, neck, trachea, esophagus, mouth, teeth, and ears as well as the cervical ganglia medulla nerve plexus
- Energizes the hypothalamus, thyroid and parathyroid; thyroxin.

Expression with clarity and integrity is an agent for progress and evolution, peace, and healing relationships.

(continued)

Basic Tenets of the Chakra System (continued)

VI Brow Chakra:

Function: Enhances quality of thought and all aspects of mind, including intuitive wisdom

Consciousness Level: Experience level

- Focuses our ability to see accurately in life, to analyze, think, reason, perceive, understand, discern, dream, imagine, and visualize
- Center of personal vision, fostering focused clarity without distortion
- Able to think in archetypes and symbols and loves the abstract and fantasy
- Hypervigilant and visually aware
- Expresses the AGAPE aspect of love
- Located at the third eye between eyebrows (green), connecting to the head, eyes, and all sense organs as well as the autonomic nervous system
- Energizes the pituitary gland; vasopressin.

This center embodies the root essence of the first five chakras and receives psychic and spiritual direction from spiritual entities.

VII Crown Chakra:

Function: Serves as the center for our highest spiritual consciousness and personal expression, connecting us to the Source of Life

Consciousness Level: Mastery level

- Opens the way for us to become a bearer of light in the world
- Focuses our attention on the spiritual meaning of life
- Begins to erase the imagined demarcation between what is spiritual and what is not
- Fosters enlightenment and self-realization
- Located at the top of head (gold), it energizes the pineal gland, brain stem, spinal cord, and CNS
- Representing "Inner Wisdom," it combines with the brow and higher octave of the throat chakra creating the Spiritual Triangle through which the three higher aspects of consciousness (wisdom, will, and activity) are expressed.

It receives psychic and spiritual energies directly from higher dimensions.

even more mysterious is the question of spirit: how does the soul move through us to guide us on our path of destiny? Where does the silent voice of our own deep knowing whisper its advice, support, and love as we move through our life journey?

Chakra Connections

Chakras are centers of awareness in the human body. These energy centers are neither physical nor anatomical, resting rather within the subtle-energy system Govinda (2009). However, their radiant energy does correspond to positions within the body. Chakras influence cells, organs, and the entire hormone system while also affecting one's thoughts and feelings. They are also centers of psychic energy. The major chakras are situated in a vertical line ascending from the base of the spine to the head.

Science of Chakras

The Chakra System, the Vital Life Force of "Prana," is a form of the Universal Energy Field. It is transformed into vitality globules, which serve the same purpose in the etheric vital body as red blood corpuscles serve in distributing oxygen to the cells of the physical body.

We are capable of feelings of great vitality and aliveness or deep fatigue and low energy. The activation of the vital blueprint is sensed as an energy movement we experience as "sensory feelings" within the physical body. This vitality can most easily be detected at certain points in the body, the chakra points. These "chakra points" are located close to a major nerve plexus and a major endocrine gland. Serving as an energy transformer, they step down the energy of one frequency to a lower level, which can be transported by specific subtle-energetic channels into the cellular structure of the physical body. At these points, vital energy is made into physical representations (Motoyama, 1981) (Figure 3.6).

These primary chakras begin as centers within the etheric body. They are connected to each other and to portions of the physical-cellular structure through fine threads of subtle energy called *nadis*. These nadis represent an extensive network of fluid-like energies that parallel bodily nerves in their abundance and function. Various sources report up to 72,000 nadis or etheric channels

FIGURE 3.6

Chakras

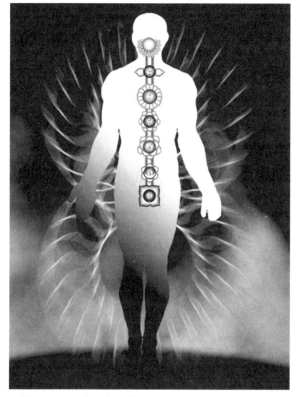

SOURCE: Adapted from B.S. Fisher (1996b), *Man, grand reflections of greater cosmic studies in occult anatomy* (Vol. 3) (Prescott, AZ: Subru Publications), p. 18.

of energy in the subtle anatomy of human beings. Interwoven with the physical nervous system, they affect the nature and quality of nerve transmission through the brain network. Dysfunction of the chakra system impacts the quality of the nervous system as well as the attached endocrine gland and nerve plexus necessary for optimal human functioning (Anodea, 2004; Govinda, 2009).

Wellness is a multidimensional phenomenon requiring homeostasis within the concrete physical body as well as a continuous flow of vital energy movement into that concrete body for a balancing of various aspects of this Prana energy. When a dynamic state of balance and harmony exist between the physical and energy aspects of our being, optimal well-being and vitality are experienced.

Soul Connection

Seed Atoms are the relatively permanent energy forms that constitute our Soul. They hold the universal archetypes, referenced by Plato and Jung (Jung, 1971; Plato, 1928;), of our individual lives (Figure 3.7).

Seed Atoms are crystal forms of spiritual anatomy, which contain all attributes and knowledge acquired through all evolutions of the consciousness cycles. Emanating from their storehouse in the Causal Body, they are implanted in the fetus during "quickening" between the 18th to 21st days of fetal development. Located at strategic points within the physical body, patterns of this life experience are impressed upon the Seed Atoms, similar to recording information on a hard drive in the computer (Fisher, 1996b, pp. 5–8).

FIGURE 3.7

Seed Crystals

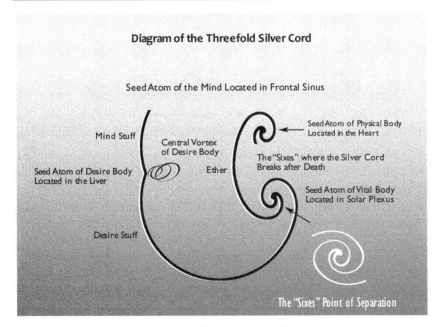

SOURCE: Adapted from B.S. Fisher (1996), *Man, grand reflection of greater cosmos: Studies in occult anatomy* (Vol.3) (Prescott, AZ: Subru Publications), p. 6.

Basic Tenets of Soul and Seed Atoms

- *The Seed Atom of the Physical Body* is located in the left ventricle of the heart. Freshly aerated blood enters from the lungs, carrying holographic pictures of all life events, taken in through the air we breathe, carried by the blood, and ultimately recorded by the permanent physical seed atom in the heart.
  Those impressions we did not consciously note—that is, were not attentive to—constitute the unconscious mind.

- *The Seed Atom of the Vital Body* is located in the solar plexus, by the spleen, capturing all modifications made to the vital blueprint throughout the lifespan.

- *The Seed Atom of the Desire/Emotional Body* is located in the central vortex of the desire/emotional body in the vicinity of the liver, recording all emotional thoughts and urges as well as higher aspirations experienced in our lived experience.

- *The Seed Atom of the Mind* is located in the frontal sinus, in the energy field surrounding the pineal gland, capturing all thoughts, ideas, and creative ventures crafted within the current life journey.

- *The Silver Cord* is the energy connection that joins the four seed atoms of our spiritual anatomy. Entering our body through the crown chakra, it flows through the CNS to the heart chakra. It serves as the connecting link between all of our bodies of consciousness, remaining attached to the physical body throughout this lifetime.

Science of Soul

The Transfer of Life Experiences occurs upon experiencing death, starting with the rupture of the seed atom of the heart. Recent life impressions stored in subconscious memory are transferred as *soul qualities* to the vital body seed atom in the solar plexus, much as we make a copy of a CD recording. The personality ego then perceives an unemotional panoramic review in reverse order, of the life ended from all stored seed atoms.

Rupture of the Silver Cord occurs upon completion of the transfer and life review. The ego becomes separated from the physical and etheric bodies and the supply of the vital Life Force is cut off, causing both bodies to disintegrate. The spiritual ego now moves in stages through the remaining energy bodies until it comes to rest in the Causal Body, with all the information and inspiration of the life encoded into the soul.

During this life experience, spiritual distress can be the originating point for physical illness. Patterns encoded in the personality and spiritual ego include both assets and shortcomings of all previous lifetimes as well as the current one. Correction of our imbalances is the goal of Personal Transformation as we grow in capacity during our lifetime. *True spiritual healing involves integration, the recovery of a sense of wholeness through the reconnection of the personality and the spirit.* Integration of ego separateness eliminates vital body imbalances due to emotional preferences, restoring balance to all bodies of consciousness. This process of "enlightenment" is referred to in esoteric healing traditions as Spiritual Alchemy (Hall, 2003).

The Causal Body serves as the spiritual repository that allows us to meld and become one with the Source. It is also the protective wrapper around our other four energy bodies, providing support, information, past life knowledge, and possibilities for our future. Spiritual Consciousness connects us to possibilities beyond those of our Soul experience. In this state, we create our own reality.

Our Spiritual Ego grows in power, wisdom, and capacity by assimilating the essence of experience gained in successive lifetimes as Soul Qualities extracted from experience in the lower bodies of form, our personality. The distillation of the essence of our bodily experiences provides the energetic nourishment for our spiritual nature to acquire permanent patterns of vibration in the Seed Atoms of the Causal Body, as the basis for personal transformation. It is also the home of Universal Spiritual Qualities such as peace and compassion, which are equally present in all human beings. As our soul growth progresses, these qualities become a natural part of who we are in the concrete world. When others experience these qualities in our personality field, our presence becomes trusted, facilitating the healing/restoration of others' own soul connection.

Dynamic Balance

Contemporary nursing practice requires two distinct functions: the clinical practice of the profession and the modeling of what we seek for others in our own life. How healthy are you? What level of vitality and well-being is present in your current life situation?

What balance is present in your life? What healing practices do you ascribe to in routines of your day?

All living systems move toward a state of stability and harmony with other systems. Because we consistently grow and change, we are in constant interchange with our environment in a disruptive way, moving in and out of balance in the perpetual dance of life. A sense of right timing and proper alignment infuses our connections and relationships with grace, filling our lives with a rhythm and harmony that is the hallmark of health.

The quantum science–based law of polarity states that from molecular to cosmic phenomena, all things exist as opposite electromagnetic fields, with a third neutral force in the center that is not accessible to direct observation or understanding. Nothing can exist except in relation to its opposite. The positive is forever transforming into the negative, whereas the negative is transforming into the positive; each power needs the other to exist. When things change, they move through a small neutral portal at the center. The emergence of new order, suggested by chaos theory, flows through this opening. When creating or managing health or change, pushing or pulling is a signal that alignment is not yet perfected. The act of honoring intuition that "senses" right timing is an essential capacity for living in balance (Koerner, 2004a, pp. 93–98).

Balance is a multifaceted diamond when viewed through the eyes of our diverse and beautiful world. A typical Western view of balance asserts that it is attained when there is physical, mental, and emotional harmony. A strong focus on physical and mental aspects of health helps us master the management of the material world and both our body and our life space.

Indigenous plains people focus on the emotional and spiritual dimensions of balance, with their emphasis on thoughts, feelings, and the manifestation of expectations. All of these things arise from deeply held beliefs and attitudes. Finding the meaning embedded within a life event is the balancing force that guides and heals.

Lakota Spiritual healer, Wanigi Waci, observed that polar opposites are the same thing in extreme, with each serving a valid function (Koerner, 2004b, pp. 121–122)

> We are spiritual beings who come to the material world for concrete human experience. We come to experience the whole spectrum of emotions: joy and sorrow, pain and pleasure, love and betrayal.

It is only by experiencing the opposites that our understanding of the phenomenon becomes whole and balanced. Each duality is the same element in differing degrees, so the key to spiritual growth resides in the ability to embrace each one fully. While the joy of friendship is meaningful, so is the sadness of tragedy. Cherish them equally and do not seek out one more than the other. When you can touch both poles with equivalent ease, you are living in harmony and balance, and the true lessons to be learned will be yours.

Balance is found when you can stand in the middle in any circumstance, with no attachment or judgment, moving freely and adaptively across the continuum.

Chinese philosophy uses the yin-yang diagram to depict balance. It suggests that the universe is run by a single principle, the Tao or Great Ultimate. This principle divides into two forces that oppose one another in their actions: yin and yang. Together they accomplish change, which emerges through the most powerful point, the yo. Intersecting between yin and yang, the yo is the refining dimension that connects these two opposing forces. This flexible space creates a *dynamic balance* rather than balance-in-the-static-leveling-out sense. Living in the flow (yo) is the optimal state of balance, achieved by moving within the dynamic center of life rather than at a single polar point (Lao-Tzu, 1992).

In his compelling book, *No Boundaries*, Ken Wilber compares a dynamic boundary to the sea. The ever-changing point of connection between land and ocean moves with the tide. He suggests that, rather than viewing a boundary as a line that keeps things in or out, the boundary can be seen as the point of connection. As we become more skilled at the subtle and immaterial realms, we can keep moving and managing the changing energy shifts in purposeful and meaningful ways (Wilber, 1985).

Exploration into the physical and spiritual domains of science and consciousness leave the nurse healer of contemporary 21st century medicine with a wide array of tools and technologies to help foster a healing experience. Models for establishing and maintaining optimal health abound and can guide nurses in their own healing practices. From a centered and holistic perspective, they can then offer guidance and support to others on their own healing journey. Further, the blending of allopathic and integrative medicine with ancient spiritual wisdom and modern faith will offer a healing model to address all levels of body/consciousness in culturally sensitive ways, transforming the health of society and the earth.

> From the cowardice that shrinks from new truth,
> From the laziness that is content with half-truths
> From the arrogance that thinks it knows all truth,
>   O God of Truth, deliver us.

An Ancient Scholar

Applying the Concepts in Nursing

You are what you believe. Some people have 1 year of life experience for 20 years, while others have 20 years of life experience. The degree to which we are open and ever learning, to that extent life is a rich adventure. Given your unique cultural, academic, and experiential background, articulate what you believe about the world today. Identify which of the concepts in this chapter resonate with familiarity and which may cause a sense of unease or pushing back.

> We are living through one of the most fundamental shifts in history—a change in the actual belief structure of Western society. No economic, political, or military power can compare with the power of a change of mind. By deliberately changing their images of reality, people are changing the world.

Willis Harman

WORLDVIEW EXERCISE

A worldview comprises the following seven components. Please consider your position on each of these questions:

1. *A Model of the World:* Who are we? Why is there something rather than nothing?
2. *An Explanation:* Why is the world the way it is? Where does it come from? How does it work?
3. *Futurology:* Where are we going? What happens to a person at death?

4. *Values:* What is evil? How do you determine right from wrong?
5. *Action:* How should we act? How do you explain human nature?
6. *Knowledge:* What is true, and what is false? How do we know what we know?
7. *Building Blocks:* What is the meaning of history? What preexisting theories and models have been used to answer the questions of the other six categories?

Checking In

What is my view of the inner and outer landscape of my life? How do I relate to them both and reconcile differences?

Balanced World View

This and That vs. Either–Or

Modern Science
- Act on Environment
  - Outer Focus
  - Predict and Control
  - Answer and Defend
  = Manage and Maintain

- Create Knowledge
  - Acquire Material Resources
  - Examine Parts
  - Count Quantity
  - Discover The Knowable
  = Physical Dimension

Living Systems
- Receive Environment
  - Inner Focus
  - Transcend and Enlarge
  - Question and Co-create
  = Becoming More

- Acquire Wisdom
  - Cultivate Relationships
  - Map Patterns
  - Experience Quality
  - Create Meaning
  = Spiritual Dimension

What do I believe constitutes the body, mind, and spirit? How do I tend—or ignore—mine each day? What would be the risk and/or reward of enlarging my view of what constitutes vibrant health? What happens to the patients I serve if I do not?

A Living Example

Naturalist John Muir, known for studying and exploring nature by living in it for extended periods of time, was frequently accompanied by his dog, Stickeen. The dog had an enduring and loyal relationship with Muir, and he liked to join Muir even in the middle of storms and in treacherous country.

On a trip across an Alaskan glacier, Muir discovered that night was falling, and he and Stickeen faced an enormous crevasse that was passable only by a precarious ice-sliver bridge. Muir realized that there was no alternative but to cross the deep and broad chasm by walking the narrow ice-covered ledge.

There was no way he could safely carry the dog across with him, so with great remorse, he left the dog behind. Stickeen watched intently as Muir walked the ledge to safety. Muir looked back at the sad and lonely dog who loved him so much. At first the dog paced back and forth, as he deliberated whether to also walk across the ledge It seemed an impossibility to Muir that the dog could make it. After much deliberation, the dog finally decided to walk across.

Amazingly, he made it! When he got safely to the other side he "ran and cried and barked and rolled about fairly hysterical in the sudden revulsion from the depth of despair to such triumphant joy. I tried to catch him and pet him and tell him how good and brave he was, but he would not be caught. He ran round and round, swirling like autumn leaves in an eddy, lay down and rolled head over heels." (Mighetto, 1986, p. 93)

The story is a reminder of how absolutely joyful it is to face a fear or unfamiliar challenge and move into another unknown and more liberating space successfully. Muir would report later that the courage and then delight of Stickeen had enlarged his life. Through him Muir saw a window into the soul of all who find inner strength and commitment to make a life altering choice and then the walk into the new land. Muir could not make the choice for the dog. He did, however, serve as an example and show him the way, modeling the successful outcome of such a choice. What sort of an example are you?

Web Site Resource: This Web site offers a framework that ties together the various aspects of a worldview: *http://pespmc1.vub.ac.be/WORLDVIEW.html*

BIBLIOGRAPHY

Anodea, J. (2004). *Eastern body, western mind: Psychology and the chakra system as a path to the self.* Sebastopol, CA: Celestial Arts.

Baylin, S. B. (1997). DNA methylation; tying it all together: Epigenetics, genetics, cell cycle, and cancer. *Science, 277*(5334), 1948–1957.

Bentov, I. (1978). *Stalking the wild pendulum*. New York: E. P. Dutton.

Bly, R. (1977). *The Kabir book*. Boston, MA: Beacon Press.

Chopra, D. (2009). *Reinventing the body, resurrecting the soul*. New York, NY: Harmony Books.

Fisher, B. S. (1996a). *Man, grand reflection of the greater cosmos: Studies in occult anatomy* (Vol. 1). Prescott, AZ: Subru Publications.

Fisher, B. S. (1996b). *Man, grand reflection of the greater cosmos: Studies in occult anatomy* (Vol. 3). Prescott, AZ: Subru Publications.

Frawley, D. (1989). *Ayurvedic healing*. Salt Lake City, UT: Passage Press.

Gerber, R. (1995). *Vibrational medicine: New choices for healing ourselves*. Santa Fe, NM: Bear & Company.

Gerber, R. (2001). *Vibrational medicine: The handbook of subtle energies*. Santa Fe, NM: Bear & Company.

Govinda, K. (2009). *A handbook of chakra healing: Spiritual practice for health, harmony, and inner peace*. Beijing, China: Konecky & Konecky

Green, B. (1999). *The elegant universe: Superstrings, hidden dimensions, and the quest for the ultimate theory*. New York, NY: Vintage Books.

Hall, M. P. (2003). *The secret teachings of all ages: An encyclopedic outline of Masonic, hermetic, Qabbalistic, and Rosicrucian symbolical philosophy*. New York, NY: Jeremy P. Tarcher/Penguin.

Jablonka, E., & Lamb, M. (1995). *Epigenetic inheritance and evolution: The Lamarckian dimension*. Oxford, UK: Oxford University Press.

Jones, P. A. (2001). *Death and methylation*. *Nature, 409,* 141–144.

Jung, C. G. (1971). In J. Campbell (Ed.), *The portable Jung chapter 6,* New York, NY: Viking Press.

Koerner, J. (2004a). Balance: Compassionate engagement in society. *Nurse Leader, 4*(1), 28–31.

Koerner, J. (2004b). *Mother heal myself: An intergenerational healing journey between two worlds*. Santa Rosa, CA: Crestport Press.

Kling, J. (2003). Put the blame on methylation. *The Scientist, 4,* 117–120.

Lao-Tzu. (1992). *Tao Te Ching: A new english version* (Stephen Mitchell, Tran.). San Francisco, CA: HarperCollins.

Laszlo, E., & Currivan, J. (2008). *Cosmos: A co-creator's guide to the whole-world*. Carlsbad, CA: Hay House.

Lipton, Bruce. (2005). *The biology of belief: unleashing the power of consciousness, matter and miracles*. Carlsbad, CA: Hay House Inc.

Mighetto, L. (1986). *Muir among the animals*. San Francisco, CA: Sierra Club.

Mindell, A. (2004). *The quantum mind and healing*. Charlottesville, VA: Hampton Roads Publishing Company.

Pert, C. (1998). *Molecules of emotion: Why you feel the way you feel*. London, UK: Simon & Schuster.

Plato. (1928). *Symposium* (A. Niehamas & P. Woodruff, Trans.). Oxford, England: Oxford University Press.

Pray, L. A. (2004). Epigenetics: Genome, meet your environment. *The Scientist,* 14–20.

Pribham, K. (1998). Autobiography in anecdote: the founding of experimental neuropsychology. In R. Bilder (Ed.), *The history of neuroscience in autobiography* (pp. 306–349). San Diego, CA: Academy Press.

Prigogine, I. (1976). Order through fluctuation: Self-organization and social system. In E. J. Jantsch & C. H. Waddington (Eds.), *Evolution and consciousness* (pp. 93–133). Reading, MA: Addison-Wesley.

Prophet, E. C., & Spadaro, P. R. (1995). *Your seven energy centers: A holistic approach to physical, emotional and spiritual vitality.* Corwin Springs, MT: Summit University Press.

Schempp, W. J. (1998). *Magnetic resonance imaging: Mathematic foundations and applications.* London, UK: Wiley-Liss.

Seppa, N. (2000). Silencing the BRCA1 gene spells trouble. *Science News,* 17, 247.

Sheldrake, R. (1981). *A new science of life.* Los Angeles, CA: Tarcher.

Silverman, P. H. (2004). Rethinking genetic determinism: With only 30,000 genes, what is it that makes humans human? *The Scientist,* 18(10), 32–33.

Svoboda, R., & Lade, A. (1995). *Tao and dharma: A comparison of Ayurveda and Chinese medicine.* Twin Lakes, WI: Lotus Press.

Szent-Gyorgyi, A. (1968). *Bioelectronics.* New York, NY: Academic Press.

Talbot, M. (1996). *The holographic universe.* London, UK: Harper Collins.

Wilber, K. (1985). *No boundary: Eastern and Western approaches to personal growth.* Boston, MA: Shambhala.

Willett, W. C. (2002). Balancing life-style and genomics research for disease prevention. *Science, 296,* 695–698.

CHAPTER 4

HEALING PRESENCE
THE PATH OF ENGAGEMENT

Do not think that love, in order to be genuine, has to be extraordinary.
What we need is to love without getting tired.
How does a lamp burn? Through the continuous input of small drops of oil.
If the drops of oil run out, the light of the lamp will cease. . . .
My daughters, what are these drops of oil in our lamps?
They are the small things of daily life;
faithfulness, punctuality, small words of kindness, a thought for others,
our way of being silent, of looking, of speaking, and of acting.
These are the true drops of love . . . .
Be faithful in small things because it is in them that your strength lies.

Mother Teresa

Many things in life matter, but only one thing really matters absolutely. It matters whether we succeed or fail in the eyes of the world. It matters whether we are healthy or not, whether we are educated or not, it matters if we are rich or poor—that certainly makes a difference in how our lives unfold. Although all of these things matter, relatively speaking, they don't matter absolutely.

There is one thing that matters more than any of those things; it is finding the essence of who we are beyond the short-lived personalized sense of self. For when we are aligned with the innate rhythms and patterns of our soul, we are in harmony with All-That-Is. Peace is not found in rearranging the circumstances of our life but, rather, by realizing who we are at the deepest level of our being (Tolle, 2003).

We are born with an insatiable curiosity and desire to learn, an instinctive drive filled with awe, wonder, and passion for discovery. Real learning that expands our understanding and our capacity involves a continuous experiment, exploring the outcome of every encounter and moving forward with the insight gained. Occasionally, we are invited to the very edge of our understanding—a place so vast that stepping beyond it will fundamentally change—everything—forever. It is a daring risk to transform our way of being in the world!

Where there is no freedom there is security; the opposite of security is *not* insecurity: *it is freedom*. Expanding our awareness requires the movement of stepping into a new space where we are totally insecure about what will happen next. Studies have shown that when children are faced with an intriguing situation and restraint from a parent, they will choose the learning experience. Not because they don't love their parents but because biological consciousness, curiosity, is stronger than love. It involves being totally ready to move outward, away from safety, even if it jeopardizes one's own life. Such is the intelligence of evolution: expanding consciousness is not possible without curiosity and learning (Schoch, 2005, p. 18). This kind of evolutionary learning is facing nursing in the postmodern world.

Health care in the 21st century requires a radically different practitioner, a nurse who must transcend the caring model that has been practiced since the discipline's inception. In her path breaking work, *Postmodern Nursing and Beyond*, nurse theorist Jean Watson (1999) addresses the changing landscape of health care in general and nursing specifically. She identified the need for nursing to not only embrace a new health care paradigm that honors the feminine but to also adopt an ontological shift of a deeper nature.

This evolutionary shift in perspective acknowledges the emerging symbiotic relationship between humankind–technology–nature and the larger, expanding universe. Declaring that a sea change of such magnitude is evoking a return to the sacred core of humanity, she invites nurses to develop a transpersonal caring focus in their practice (Watson, pp. 290–291).

> Transpersonal conveys a human connection, beyond personal body-physical ego, and has a spiritual dimension; it implies a focus on the uniqueness of self and other coming together, moving from the fully embodied physical ego-self to deeper, more

spiritual, transcendent even cosmic connections that tap into healing; transpersonal includes the unique individuality of each human, while extending beyond the ego-self, radiating and transcending to deeper connections all humans share with their deeper selves, the other, environment, nature and the universe.

Transpersonal caring is a founding construct for the essence of a healing presence. This stance will bring nursing from the modern into the postmodern era, giving us the opportunity to reinstate the sacred feminine into the healing arts. Restoring the masculine–feminine balance will return the possibility for wholeness to the healing experience. As all health care workers incorporate methods that work directly with cycle, rhythm, resonance, reciprocity, and right relationship—the patterns of the feminine—the power of the self to heal will be potentiated. As dynamic balance and respect return, cooperative and collaborative holistic practice models will increasingly emerge. And the way that care is provided and experienced will be transformed.

BEING WITH—THE SPIRITUAL DIMENSION OF NURSING

Nursing is a relational phenomenon. Everything we see, everything we do, and everything we experience arises out of a *relationship*: to people and their families of cultures rich and varied, to physiology strong or failing, to colleagues of many disciplines, to communities in stress, to a world seeking to find its way. The only constant in this multidimensional world we serve is ourSelf.

The privilege of being a nurse gives us multiple opportunities for expansive and co creative relationships that enlarge our capacities and sensibilities. To partner with society in their quest for health deliberately and with compassion is the call for authentic nurses. These nurses know their own worldview while appreciating and drawing on the view of others. Although they understand illness and institutional caring, they are equally at home in roles fostering health within every sector of society.

Noted quantum physicist Dana Zohar made a startling discovery (1990). After the birth of her daughter, she became a mother. She then had a son and found that she was a different being. The role and responses in the relationship were decidedly different from the one shared with her daughter. She concluded that, like the elements in quantum physics, we are a quantum self. If we show up authentically and engage in the moment, we cocreate our reality with another, just as particles and waves cocreate the Universe. The more genuine relationships we engage in, the more dimensions emerge in our personality and consciousness. There is no limit to the endless variations and iterations of "self" that reside in each of us if we remain an open system, hovering with flexibility on the edge of chaos.

Nursing is the unifying element in the clinical and spiritual care offered to people in a health crisis. We are the sentinel at the bedside during the moment of birth, death, and every conceivable scenario in between. Each day we are privileged to witness and support the suffering of a fellow traveler on this daunting earth journey. We engage with their issues, gaining strength and wisdom ourselves from their unique moments of courage and brokenness as they gather up the broken fragments of their life. With compassionate nonjudgment, we support their movement toward a revised version of health or to a peaceful death.

What is "it" that we offer that makes a difference? How do we touch their experience in a manner that is helpful and hopeful, that is healing rather than diminishing? Or, do we? Modern nursing has been so flooded with information, technology, and documentation demands that the very reason we go into nursing—to be within service—is often no longer experienced by the person or ourselves. Intentionally practicing the spiritual dimension of nursing creates a safe and compassionate space that allows others to sort through their situation honestly, clearly, with candor and courage. This moment of chaos in their lives is meant to help them discover what is no longer working, what they have outgrown, and turn their gaze toward a revised way of living that is enlarging to their life. Our healing presence offers the sanctuary needed for that kind of soul work.

From a stance of reverence and openness toward limitless possibilities, we bring the spiritual aspect of our being into our nursing practice and our relationships with others. Before we can offer such a perspective to others, we must first cultivate spiritual consciousness within ourselves. However, the call for this transpersonal awareness is not a call to sainthood; it is a call to *authenticity*.

In their compelling book *The Spirituality of Imperfection*, Kurtz and Ketcham compare the discovery of spirituality to playing baseball, the only sport that considers errors to be an integral part of the game (1992, p. 1):

> *Spirituality teaches us, or has taught most of us, how to deal with failure.* We learn at a very young age that failure is the norm in life . . . errors are part of the game, part of its rigorous truth.

For thousands of years, every day saints and mystics have explored the ordinary and common in an attempt to understand the extraordinary and divine. Their various attempts call forth the spiritual realities of humility, gratitude, tolerance, and forgiveness. The spirituality of imperfection begins with the recognition that trying to be perfect is the most tragic human mistake. When we cease trying to be perfect, by embracing our errors and shortcomings and accepting that we cannot control every aspect of our lives, we begin to find peace and serenity and the joy of our authentic selves. This sense of an imperfect reality is what we offer to those we support in their own less-than-perfect moment as they sort through the illness crisis.

For us individually, and nursing as a collective, to move deeper into our own being and then extending it as an offering to others requires the courage to see the truth of what is: To be totally present, to simply observe what is there, and establish a relationship with it. We will discover that within ourselves, and in each human being, there is a dimension of consciousness far deeper than thought; it is the *essence of who we are*. It has been referred to as many things including presence, awareness, unconditional consciousness, the Christ within, or your Buddha nature (Hollick, 2006).

Finding that dimension frees us, and the world, from the suffering that we inflict upon ourselves through the countless little judgments made by the ego personality that runs our lives. Love, peace, and creativity cannot be heard while that deeply conditioned dimension of consciousness dominates. When we step out of the content of our lower mind, the incessant stream of thinking slows down. Thoughts don't absorb all of our attention anymore. Gaps arise in between thoughts—spaciousness—stillness. In the silence, we begin to realize how much vaster and deeper we are than our random and programmed thoughts. The door to our inner world begins to open.

As our self-awareness grows, we can recognize, even for a second, that the thoughts running through our mind are simply thoughts, habits, and patterns that do nothing except divert our attention and energy toward maintaining the status quo. The human mind, with its curious drive to know, understand, and control, mistakes its own opinions and viewpoints as the truth. It continually tells us "this is how it is," and we believe it.

Expanded consciousness, our Spiritual Ego, which is larger than thought, helps us to realize that no matter how we interpret our life or the life or behavior of another, it's no more than a point of view, one of many possible perspectives. Thinking fragments reality into conceptual bits and pieces. But the perspective of soul sees the subtle truth that reality is one beautiful and unified whole in which all things are interwoven; nothing exists alone. From a stance of unconditional regard, we experience the union and security of being part of All-That-Is, fostering a sense of safety and peace beyond understanding. Only when we are in this loving space of oneness with all will true wisdom emerge as we "see" and "understand" holistically (Rasha, 2003).

As professionals we have been socialized to use a highly sophisticated conceptually oriented and analytical mind. Although this is a very useful and powerful tool, it is also very limiting when it overshadows our larger perspective, when we quit realizing that it is only one small aspect of the abstract wisdom in higher consciousness that we are. The curing paradigm is prescriptive, requiring the practitioner to identify what is wrong and take steps to fix it. When health is viewed as a disruption in multiple levels of energy/consciousness, the approach of treating a person with a specific intervention becomes a problem. Physician Rachel Naomi Remen observed (Kuthumi, 1996, p. 158):

> The curing relationship is not always healthy for the client. While benefiting in some ways by the relationship, the client may also be diminished because it is a dependent relationship. There is not much room for strength or growth in the kind of curing relationship that we are taught in professional schools. We can fix the fixable and direct and control specific outcomes, but we don't evoke healing, and we don't participate in the healing that may arise naturally. The fixing relation assumes that healing occurs naturally, following its own natural course. This is wrong, and the outcome is often incomplete.

Postmodern Nursing demands the best of our history as well as the embracing of an emerging future. Facilitating an open and safe environment that prompts the apprehension of wholeness is the receptive feminine function in the universe—and the core of nursing. "Seeing" the object as well as the background that holds it gives one a sense of "the whole." Ironically, as the healing fields have progressed scientifically, we have started to put our science—in the form of diagnostic labels and predictive pathways—in front of the patient/object. Standards and protocols have overshadowed the patient as our conditioning for evidence-based care has infused our practice.

The postmodern paradigm takes us back to right order: begin with the relationship to understand the "person/object" and THEN bring in the scientific background and protocols to provide care. This requires the nurse to bring her *authentic presence* to the relationship, starting at the *point of nonintervention.*

Tenet of Authentic Healing Presence

The Postmodern Nursing Paradigm focused on healing is relationship based not intervention focused:

- Awareness and presence are the initiating mechanisms for establishing an authentic relationship.
- Authentic healing relationship fosters a co creative partnership based on respect and trust.
- Nursing science and clinical intervention reside in the background, waiting to be brought forward for use as determined by information gained in the relationship rather than the chart or diagnosis.
- Nonintervention is based on principles of holographic wave interference:
  - Concentric rings of light energy, originating primarily in the heart chakra, create an individual wave pattern unique to each individual.
  - Energy waves are holographic in nature, with an image of the whole written on each part.
  - As waves radiate toward each other, they meet and interact, forming an interference pattern.

(continued)

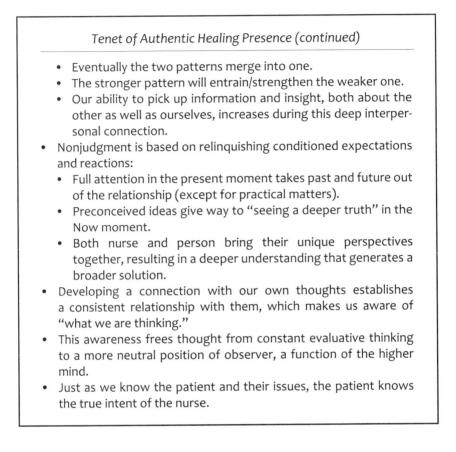

Tenet of Authentic Healing Presence (continued)

- Eventually the two patterns merge into one.
- The stronger pattern will entrain/strengthen the weaker one.
- Our ability to pick up information and insight, both about the other as well as ourselves, increases during this deep interpersonal connection.
- Nonjudgment is based on relinquishing conditioned expectations and reactions:
  - Full attention in the present moment takes past and future out of the relationship (except for practical matters).
  - Preconceived ideas give way to "seeing a deeper truth" in the Now moment.
  - Both nurse and person bring their unique perspectives together, resulting in a deeper understanding that generates a broader solution.
- Developing a connection with our own thoughts establishes a consistent relationship with them, which makes us aware of "what we are thinking."
- This awareness frees thought from constant evaluative thinking to a more neutral position of observer, a function of the higher mind.
- Just as we know the patient and their issues, the patient knows the true intent of the nurse.

SCIENCE OF HEALING PRESENCE

We are called to move from beginning the nurse–patient connection with a diagnosis and intervention focus, to coming into an authentic relationship with no mind. When we place a label on a person or situation, we confuse the conditioned mind maps and plans with the truth of what is before us. To function in this way is an unconscious pattern, deeply conditioned through childhood, cultural, and professional socialization. Once we place a conceptual identity on something, it becomes a prison for both the other and for ourselves.

When we give our full attention to the present moment and what we are interacting with, we take past and future out of the relationship, except for practical matters. Immediate and emergent conditions always demand a swift response, however. As we relinquish conditioned expectations and reactions, attention steps in and shows us a deeper truth, making the resulting intervention more profound and therapeutic. In the process, both the nurse and the person increase their awareness and understanding from the unique perspective that is their own. Both come away from the exchange with an enlarged knowing but in different and unique ways appropriate for their own issues and capacities.

The scientific nursing process is well known; it is the foundation of our practice. As we bring transpersonal dimensions of practice into our work, a paradox occurs. While managing clinical diagnosis and interventions, we must simultaneously practice in *the realm of nonintervention*. We cannot know what form the multidimensional pattern of a person will take as their awareness expands. Therefore, the new paradigm that focuses on healing is relational in nature. The nurse and patient enter into a partnership, an authentic relationship where both persons trust the process that evolves. This requires the nurse to bring her awareness and presence, rather than her clinical protocols, as the *initiating* mechanism for establishing a therapeutic relationship. Of course, the science and interventions of professional practice are always there, but they reside in the background, waiting to be called upon, rather than in the foreground controlling what is trying to emerge.

> Placing nursing/caring into a spiritual perspective in no way diminishes what we have to offer others through training, experience, individuality, special skills, or sense of the humane. Quite the reverse. Our particular talents and unique qualities are likely to come forth more reliably when we do have a richer and more spacious sense of who we are—the very promise of all spiritual practice.
>
> *Ram Dass*

Nonintervention is based on a holographic model of wave interference. Concentric rings of light energy are consistently emanating from every living thing. In the human, they originate in the heart chakra, primarily, and other chakras secondarily (Djwal Kul, 1996). (Figure 4.1)

Each person has a specific wave pattern that reflects their personality/consciousness and the vibrational capacity of their bioenergetic body. Energy waves are holographic in nature, with

FIGURE 4.1

Energy Vibrations Emanating From Chakras

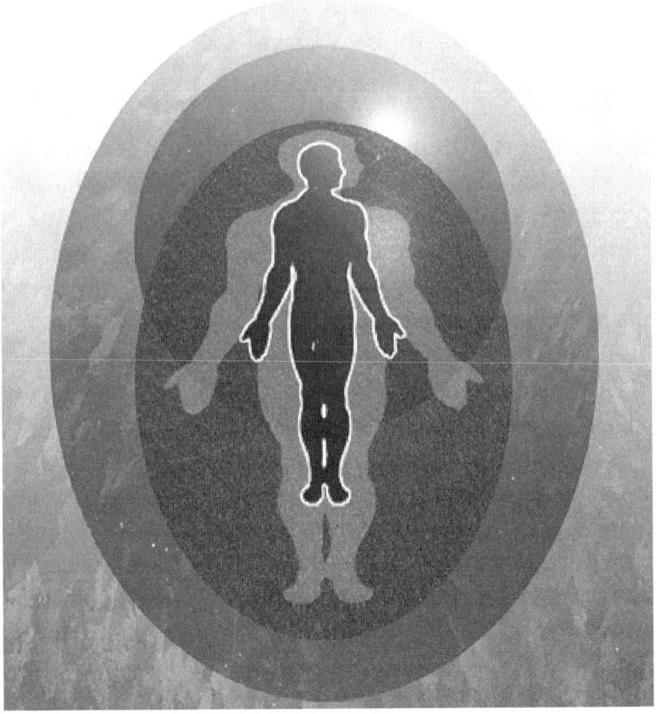

the image of the whole written on each part, so all is known when a merging of consciousness fields occurs.

Just as waves emerge from two pebbles tossed into water, energy waves are emitted from two people in close proximity. As the waves radiate toward each other, they meet and interact, and an interference pattern evolves. The pattern spreads and is part of the whole of the two previous patterns as they merge into one (Figure 4.2). Just as the nurse "senses into" the patient and recognizes their patterns, so too, the person senses into the nurse and "feels" their own patterns and attitudes. Indifference, frustration, and fatigue on the part of the nurse are recognized by the person, who often infers that the nurse is "not interested in me." To intentionally be in touch with the other person and the environment, one must be in touch with their own pattern.

FIGURE 4.2

Interference Patterns Between Two Persons

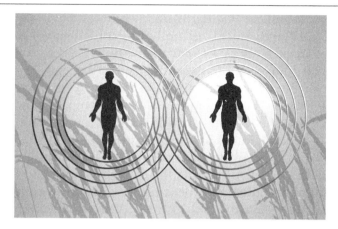

Research has shown that when two people focus on each other in a meaningful way, their EEG patterns merge as one. Our ability to pick up signals increases during a deep interpersonal connection. Braud's research further demonstrated that the most ordered brain pattern always prevailed. Mental and physical structures of a highly organized person exerted an ordering influence on the less-organized recipient (Braud, 2000). (Figure 4.3)

FIGURE 4.3

Two Patterns Merging as One

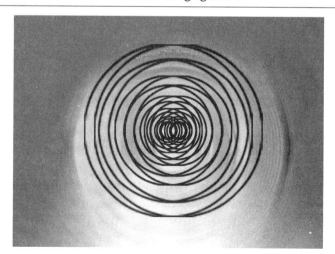

Interference Patterns Between Two Persons

The person and nurse are interpenetrating aspects of a shared whole. The unbroken wholeness of this partnership is also part of the Universal Energy Field, as the holographic view of the world is enfolded in each region of space-time. Individual pattern is contained within our own orb, while in nested fashion, in a shared space we become part of another. On the Universal level, we are part of All-That-Is. The order recorded in the complex movement of these electromagnetic fields enfolds the entire information of the universe in each region of space and time (Bohm, 1981). The better we know ourselves, the more clearly we "sense into" other persons as well as information from the collective field, and the more meaningful our relationships become. The highest form of knowing is love, the essence of the Spirit of Universal Consciousness. Vibrational frequency at that level creates a sense of oneness.

A nurse who is authentically present moves between the world of clinical practice and the context of the person's life (ground), weaving an invisible web of interconnection between the immediate and the important, between the visible and the invisible, between endings and beginnings, between despair and renewal. This vibrant space of all possibility gives the person safety, perspective, hope, and direction for the life that is emerging out of the chaos of the health event.

To see and respond to the invisible half of wholeness, nursing must expand its capacity in all three domains of the Triad of Compassionate Caring: the science, the art, and the presence of their practice. The "evaluator aspect" of the nurse as scientist must develop the mechanisms of *active observation*. The "interpreter aspect" of the nurse as artist must increase skills in *active intelligence*. And, the "witness aspect" of the presence of the nurse must increase the capacity to create and maintain a context of *active receptivity*, the space that integrates all with spiritual ego. Building on the strong framework for practice, which is our heritage, we must now make the "quantum leap" into a new dimension if we are to honor our social commitment to the public we are privileged to serve.

The notion of "active" implies *an enlarging awareness* coming from a place *beyond the thinking mind*. Judgment and labels, prejudice of any kind, imply that we are identified with the thinking mind. It means that we don't see the other human being any longer, only our predetermined concept of that person. To reduce the aliveness of another to a concept or diagnosis is a form of violence.

Thinking that is not rooted in awareness becomes self-serving and dysfunctional. Intelligence devoid of wisdom is extremely dangerous and destructive (as seen in the prevalence of war in today's society). Focus coming from the thinking mind is the current state of mass consciousness in humanity. The amplification of thought as science and technology, though not intrinsically good or bad, has become destructive because so often the thinking out of which it arises has no roots in awareness.

Nursing in the postmodern world must move from thinking to the stance of wisdom. Wisdom is not a product of thought. The deep *knowing* that is wisdom arises through the simple act of giving someone or something your full attention. Attention is primordial intelligence, consciousness itself. This powerful awareness dissolves the barriers created by conceptual thought, and with this comes the recognition that nothing exists by itself. It joins the perceiver and that which is perceived into a unified field of awareness (Tolle, 2003, p. 16). *It is the energy of conscious awareness, ushered in through a healing presence, which invites and honors the deep wisdom of the soul to initiate the healing process within one's self.*

ACTIVE OBSERVATION—SEEING BEYOND THE OBVIOUS

Clinical assessment is the foundation for nursing practice. Once the therapeutic relationship is established, the task set before the nurse is to "evaluate" the phenomenon at hand from an objective stance and then create a plan of care. The patient experience is dictated by the depth and breadth of the assumptions, observations, and conclusions drawn by the nurse about their situation. Patient care needs addressed will include only the things that our awareness and understanding can recognize. The patient is at the mercy of the nurse.

The focus of our current professional education curriculum has been on "clinical assessment," evaluating the status of the body and the emotional/spiritual well-being of the person entrusted to our care. In the postmodern world, an expanded approach is required of the nurse healer. Assessing the entire human bioenergy

Tenet of Active Observation

Active Observation—Scientific Role of Nurse as Evaluator

- Passive Mechanism of "Looking"
  - Energy patterns of light radiate from the object observed.
  - Light carries information about its form and focuses through refraction on the retina of the eye.
  - This pattern is transmitted by light-sensitive cells (rods and cones) via the optic nerve onto the physical brain.
- Active Mechanism of "Seeing"
  - Like a radar system, an energy stream is emitted by the optic nerve and beamed through the "third eye" located by the brow chakra onto the object being observed.
  - Beam illuminates and penetrates the object and mingles with the energy pattern of the object as interference patterns meet in holographic fashion, wrapping around the whole of the object and gathering information about the "essence of the object."
- Information is reflected back to the etheric lens of the third eye located near the brow chakra, which connects with the filter of intuition and inner wisdom.
- "Integrated Vision" provides nurse with insight into phenomenon observed:
  - Seven components link logic and intuition to create insight:
    - Eye—organ of sight that takes in light
    - Third Eye—organ of energy perception, which emits light that wraps around object observed, gathering energy patterns that stimulate intuition and inner wisdom
    - Analytic Lower Mind—discriminates and evaluates signals from eye, brain, and bodily senses, generating information
    - Abstract Higher Mind—integrates concrete data with etheric perceptions and translates them into a recognizable pattern, creating a flash of intuitive insight
    - Brain—organ of transfer that gathers and stores data
    - Intuition—"Inner Wisdom" that holds collective knowledge of all lived experiences as patterned perceptions
    - Body-Mind—control tower that takes in information as Focal Point shifts between Higher and Lower Mind to create a plan of action for the human experience.

field requires a different way of seeing; we must learn to use additional innate capacities to practice the art of active observation. Combining sight (physical vision) with perception (mental vision) creates an integrated body of knowledge to guide clinical practice.

Science of Active Observation

Moving from observation of concrete, material reality to the active surveillance of subtle energy requires the development of capacity to assess both the tangible and the subtle. It also requires us to enter the experience from a perspective of relationship rather than an interventional viewpoint. We must be open to what is *before* us—just as it is—before programmed labels and expectations are placed into the scene.

In the quantum world, we use both a passive mechanism of "looking" and an active mechanism of "seeing" to comprehend the whole of the situation under review. The "nurse evaluator" will use seven components that serve as a link between the body-mind and ego personality embedded in our body and the abstract mind and spiritual ego that reside in our soul.

There are two mechanisms used to create "integrated vision" (Fisher, 1996, pp. 49–53):

- *A Passive Mechanism*: Energy patterns in the form of light and etheric 'atoms' emanate from the object to be perceived. Light carries information about its form, focused by refracting media onto the retina of the physical eye. This pattern is transmitted by light sensitive cells (rods and cones) via the optic nerve onto the physical brain. Ordinary sight (physical vision) is based on highly organized and localized organs of perception, specialized from chemical and physical matter. This organic process helps us 'see' in the traditional sense of sight.
- *An Active Mechanism*: Likened to a radar system. An energy beam emitted by the Optic Nerve illuminates and penetrates the object to be perceived, mingles with the energy patterns emitted by the object as interference patterns meet, is reflected back, and focused on the etheric lens of the "third eye" located near the brow chakra. The energy pattern carried is impressed directly upon the Optic Disc and transmitted via the Optic Nerve onto the physical brain.

Sight (physical vision) is highly focused and concrete, whereas Perception (mental vision) is less localized and more symmetrically distributed over the ovoid surface of the emotional body and mental body auras. They each contain force centers or vortices, which function as receptors for perception of energy patterns that connect with the filters of intuition and inner wisdom. When merged together, we are given a "sense perception" of an invisible whole behind the specific object viewed by the third eye.

Along with visual assessment, we use auditory sound to deepen our understanding; we tune in to the "stereo sound" that informs a deeper knowing. When we casually focus our attention on what is being said, we "hear" the message of the words. However, when we "listen" with full attention, the vibrational level rises to the level of soul, which is sound sensitive. Our thought body senses the energetic tone, holographically perceiving the emotional messages behind the words. Giving ourselves completely to the act of listening beyond the sounds uncovers something greater, a sacredness that cannot be understood through thought (Tolle, 1999, p. 77).

ACTIVE INTELLIGENCE—KNOWING BEYOND CONCRETE THOUGHT

The art of nursing is the hallmark of our profession. Being able to step into any relationship and uncover what is uniquely important to the person, weave into a standardized plan of care, and give customized service are truly creative acts! Nurse as artist assumes the "interpreter role" as she takes the client into unknown territory with grace and ease. Much as a naturalist guide in the wilderness, she identifies points of interest as well as potential danger zones. She interprets the culture and the language, dress mores, and rituals that will be seen and encountered. Equally important, in her role as advocate she represents the client to the staff in reciprocal fashion so that, in the end, there are no strangers here.

An excellent naturalist knows the terrain, the dangers and delights, the weather patterns and where resources lie. This level of familiarity helps them anticipate challenges before they arise. A deep knowing of the landscape makes workarounds simple when one venue is closed. And by being in harmony with the animals and nature elements who reside in those climes, there is a rhythm and cadence to moving in and through the landscape.

In this new post-modern world, the Nurse Artist must engage with another dimension of reality in the nurse-patient situation: the Inner World (Dosse, Guzzetta & Kolkmeier, 1995). In truth, it has always been there, but we are just waking up to recognize it so that the totality of the person is served. This wilderness of "Inner World" is largely a mystery to both the person and the nurse; neither is fully aware of what lies within their own. Each has surprises and delights to discover, as well as dangers to transverse. The Interpreter must help guide the discovery process as they both walk to their inner truth in a way that facilitates the healing process. For the nurse to help navigate this journey successfully she must practice the art of Active Intelligence.

As information, and the world it represents, becomes more complex, nurses must move from concrete thinking (logic, analysis and understanding) to also consider the higher perspective of active intelligence which also incorporates abstract thinking (intent, intuition and wisdom). Simultaneously, we must develop the capacity to shift our Focal Point of thought from the lower dimension of body-mind-ego information to also include the higher dimension of the Spiritual Ego and Universal Wisdom. This fosters integrated intelligence, which opens up a whole new world of unending possibility.

Tenets of Active Intelligence

Active Intelligence-Artistic Role of Nurse as Interpreter between two worlds

- Human Intelligence system is divided into levels of increasing vibration
- Region of Concrete Analytic Thought (Lower Mind)
  - Home of the Body-Mind
  - *Experience is the gateway into the Body-Mind*
  - Vibrations are so low that energy is converted to form
  - Embodied thought manifests in the body as three lowest vibration levels:
    - Senses (from vital etheric body to body sensors; sight/touch and so on)
    - Feelings (from desire emotional body)
    - Experience (Home of Lower Mind "Common Sense," Personality & Ego)

(continued)

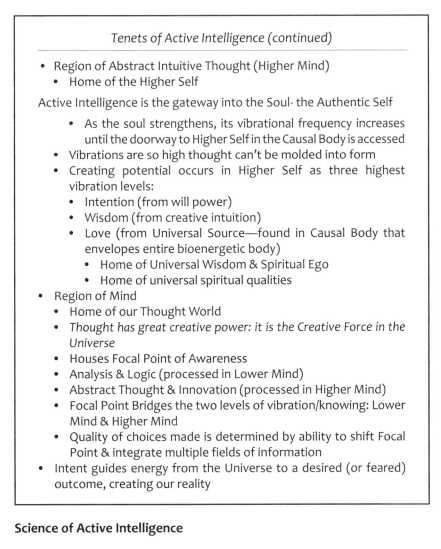

Tenets of Active Intelligence (continued)

- Region of Abstract Intuitive Thought (Higher Mind)
  - Home of the Higher Self

Active Intelligence is the gateway into the Soul- the Authentic Self

- As the soul strengthens, its vibrational frequency increases until the doorway to Higher Self in the Causal Body is accessed
- Vibrations are so high thought can't be molded into form
- Creating potential occurs in Higher Self as three highest vibration levels:
  - Intention (from will power)
  - Wisdom (from creative intuition)
  - Love (from Universal Source—found in Causal Body that envelopes entire bioenergetic body)
    - Home of Universal Wisdom & Spiritual Ego
    - Home of universal spiritual qualities
- Region of Mind
  - Home of our Thought World
  - *Thought has great creative power: it is the Creative Force in the Universe*
  - Houses Focal Point of Awareness
  - Analysis & Logic (processed in Lower Mind)
  - Abstract Thought & Innovation (processed in Higher Mind)
  - Focal Point Bridges the two levels of vibration/knowing: Lower Mind & Higher Mind
  - Quality of choices made is determined by ability to shift Focal Point & integrate multiple fields of information
- Intent guides energy from the Universe to a desired (or feared) outcome, creating our reality

Science of Active Intelligence

A nurse-healer in the postmodern world utilizes new models for discernment that transcend understanding, expanding the scholarly practice of their trade. To efficiently do this we are called to shift our Focal Point, the point of awareness, to the higher realm of abstract thought. Exploring various knowledge systems and the classical metaphysical archetypes, we come to understand a way of knowing that transcends our current knowledge systems.

The Universal Energy Field exists as the pure energy of Universal Intelligence. Energy follows subtle thought, flowing from the Universal Field housed in our Causal Body into the bioenergetic fields of our Higher Self. As a cascade of flowing energy surrounds and infuses our bioenergetic body, it swirls and moves in vibratory dance, coalescing and releasing as external influences and inner emotions and desires attract and slow it to the point of manifestation. This form of light 'impacts our body' in multiple ways as we navigate the Outer World. We acquire various levels of information, consider its meaning for us, and make a choice that leads to action. No two human beings are alike; the same energy will have different meaning and effect on two people in the same situation. What we focus on and how we interpret its meaning is a singular function. We each create and live in our own universe!

The home of human awareness, our Thought World is comprised of seven levels which are divided into two regions and a transitional mid-level (Fisher, 1996, pp. 49–53). The Mid (4th) Reflective-Mental Body serves as a bridge between our Inner (Higher) World and Outer (Lower) World; it is central to the creation and interpretation of our lived experience.

The energy anatomy of the Reflective-Mental Body is an organized cloud of force-matter; energy that is coalescing in various levels of vibratory rate in response to activities of the mind. Ovoid in shape, it encircles the head and shoulders, incorporating aspects of the physical/vital and emotional bodies, as well as providing a doorway into the Higher Mind. This amazing 'decision-making zone' holds two levels of vibration (coming from both inner and outer worlds), serving as an integrating platform for both analytic and abstract thought—if we choose to utilize both by shifting the Focal Point between the two worlds.

● Its sector of lower vibration (Lower Mind) serves as our organ of *logical thought*, our vehicle for concrete thinking. Because of our predominant, and often conditioned, thought patterns, the Focal Point's primary reference rests here, directing most of the mental body's force-matter to the brain in the physical body, which records the ongoing thoughts and emotions of the personality; the "i." A diffused and less conditioned consciousness, it creates a small 'envelope' identified strongly with our emotions and ego. Focusing on this dimension of awareness limits capacity and options, and we easily getting entangled in the external world. This aspect of the analytic mind predominates in most people today; it is mass consciousness.

- Its sector of more rapid vibration (Higher Mind) serves as a vehicle for *abstract thought*, the seat of the intuitive mind and higher intellect; the "I." It serves as the doorway into the abstract world of our Spiritual Ego. It is also the portal through which creative, germinal ideas flow from the field of infinite possibility into our higher consciousness when focused and quiet. Moral integrity resides here.
- The *home of the Soul*, connected to our individual Spirit—spark of life—residing in our Causal Body, is found within the sector of higher vibration located in the sixth dimension directly over the heart chakra. When the focal point shifts into Higher Mind, the mental body's force-matter begins to move into the world of abstract thought. The Soul, which holds the blueprint for our destiny, increasingly contributes aspects of our unique potential into our choices and lived experience. Its increased vibratory contribution also triggers our Intuition, which holds the total knowledge accumulated over this lifetime. With further development, Inner Wisdom, which is the summary of many lifetimes, is also tapped to guide our life choices and activities into the destiny we are here to experience. This increased vibrational shift and information from our Soul initiates synchronicity into our life.

When our Focal Point of reference rests in our Higher Mind, the analytic world is still available, but the initiating thoughts begin at a higher, more abstract level of consciousness. From this perspective, an active, versus. prescriptive intelligence navigates multiple dimensions and opens limitless possibilities. *In this world we co create reality rather than conform to it.*

Thought has great creative power; it is the creative force in the Universe. Creativity is a specialized way of thinking. Situational creativity, rearrangement of things that exist, is utilized as we work through issues and opportunities on a daily basis. Foundational creativity, however, is more rare and difficult. The domain of artists, adepts, and cultural creatives, it involves the creation of new order, whether in form, the written word, or social order.

The *creative act begins with focused intent.* Don Juan instructed Carlos Castaneda with these words (1972, p. 3):

> In the universe there is an immeasurable, indescribable force which shamans call intent, and absolutely everything that exists in the entire cosmos is attached to intent by a connecting link. When those who live with the Source beckon with intent, it comes to

them and sets up the path for attainment, which means they always accomplish what they set out to do.

The *field of intent guides energy from the Universe*. Nonlocal and ubiquitous, it is everywhere. This invisible and formless field is manifest in every part of our body, soul and the reality we create. It is the subtle pull toward the potential for the purpose of our life prompted by our Spiritual Ego (Woody, 2004, p. 59). When personality ego dominates, however, the power of intent is disconnected, and we become passive, living in reactive fashion in the world of our personality.

Conversely, when intent is resolute, a sincere act of will emanating from the highest aspect of our Spiritual Ego, it calls forth a concept or germinal idea which moves into the region of our Thought World. Here the thought-form attracts force-matter to create a "desire element" which will impel action in the physical world.

We may request one thing yet experience something quite different from our expectation because manifestation occurs in relation to our vibrational capacity. Thought forms follow the subtle energy patterns which radiate from our body-mind. A neutral force, they are without judgment. They honor what we are thinking about, not what we are talking about. *It is the desire/emotional body patterns that create the form of our reality.* Fear and anger are two vibrational energetic patterns that most often sabotage the longings of our heart.

Nurse-healers can strengthen and expand their Mental-Reflective capacity for Active Intelligence through disciplines of logic such as studying the new physical quantum sciences and mathematics. Focusing on artistic expressions of music and poetry, photography and stories, increases sensitivity to the subtle realm in all things. Aesthetic creative activities, noble ideas and acts of compassion increase the capacity for love-wisdom. Flexibility and adaptability increase through the practice of various forms of body work. And we can become infinitely more responsive to the subtle promptings of our own body-mind-spirit by managing emotions or cultivating the art of stillness through meditation and awareness practices.

Shifting the Focal Point requires raising our vibration, which raises the vibrations of the mental body to engage in higher mind. This makes intelligence more luminous, organizing it into a more definitive structure, freeing it from the influences of desire and emotions. Residing in higher mind makes us invulnerable to the negative and destructive thought-forms and desires created by others. Lower vibrational fields abound in the environment and are often unknowingly assimilated by us, manifesting similar negative tendencies in ourselves.

As we move the focus of our mental body toward our higher intelligence a new knowledge that transcends thought and understanding is ours. Regarding the process and its timing, Hicks (2006, p. 103) observed:

> Well-being is the only order of the day, unless you are doing something to pinch it off. So, little by little, more and more, people begin to feel comfortable with their own thoughts; especially, understanding that thoughts don't have instant manifestational power anyway. You live in this time/space reality where there is a buffer zone between the offering of a thought and the receiving of the manifestation. So it gives you a lot of opportunity to amend and add to.

As our energy pattern increases and our understanding of thought-created reality increases, everything shifts! The heavy screen of our past, concepts and attitudes through which all things were filtered, drop away. We begin to see without interpreting. From the realm of higher consciousness we can perceive the essence of what we observe (Tolle, 2005). Michelangelo remarked that "every beauty which is seen here below by persons of perception resembles more than anything else that celestial source from which we all came (Dwyer, 2004, p. 1). Increasingly we become that which we appreciate, and our healing presence unfolds as a flower responding to the first spring rain.

ACTIVE RECEPTIVITY—BEING PRESENT WITH AUTHENTICITY

Subtle energy always follows thought, while soul qualities follow love. Love, in its most universal sense, is not an emotion. Love is a state of being infused with a deep awareness of the interconnection of All-That-Is. We recognize the truth that we are One and all barriers dissolve; a deep reciprocity emerges between the person and the nurse. It is not a movement of action: love is a stance of just being there. Loving ourselves is in fact the movement of loving others. As we stand as witness for the other in an environment of love we see 'all there is'; strengths, qualities and weaknesses alike. As we stay in touch with what comes up, we identify the beauty of everything without judgment. We radiate compassion. Bearing witness to something and staying with it is the process of transpersonal caring. Whenever there is love, there is healing and transformation (Schoch, 2005).

Tenets of Active Receptivity

III-Active Receptivity: Healing Presence--Role of Nurse as Witness

- Essence is the invisible energy quality radiating from our vibrational field
  - Essence of Body is cell vibration creating electro-chemical movement that generates the *light aura* radiating around the body
  - Essence of Mind is movement of brain cells creating *mental aura* transmitting essence of our thoughts radiating out from body-mind
  - Essence of Being is the level of energy vibration of out-of-body consciousness we currently resonate which radiates a *quality aura* felt as our Presence, much like a weather pattern in the outer world
- Core Self—Spirit--is our Divine Spark of Life
  - Highest vibrational energy spectrum in humankind
  - Direct extension of the Source, unique to each of us
  - At this level we experience oneness and unity with All
  - It is housed in the Causal Body
  - It embodies Universal Spiritual Qualities such as love, compassion, and peace—residing in each human Spirit
  - As we develop our spiritual capacities, these qualities are infused into our soul in proportion to our capacity to hold that vibrational energy
- Soul holds the seed crystal of our destiny and life purpose
  - Located in energy vortex of heart chakra
  - Connects directly to our Spark of Life in the Causal Body
  - Increasingly incorporates Universal Spiritual Qualities such as love, compassion and peace, as the Spiritual Ego matures
  - Offers unique potential within us to accomplish life purpose when we access our Higher Mind
  - Seat of our 'Inner Wisdom' where we can experience our true intelligence as well as our conscience which guides moral behavior
  - Intuition is the gateway into this Inner Wisdom
  - Integration of body-mind knowledge and Inner Wisdom gives us a holistic perspective

(continued)

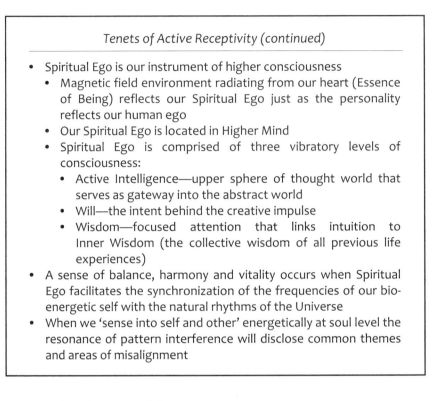

Tenets of Active Receptivity (continued)

- Spiritual Ego is our instrument of higher consciousness
  - Magnetic field environment radiating from our heart (Essence of Being) reflects our Spiritual Ego just as the personality reflects our human ego
  - Our Spiritual Ego is located in Higher Mind
  - Spiritual Ego is comprised of three vibratory levels of consciousness:
    - Active Intelligence—upper sphere of thought world that serves as gateway into the abstract world
    - Will—the intent behind the creative impulse
    - Wisdom—focused attention that links intuition to Inner Wisdom (the collective wisdom of all previous life experiences)
- A sense of balance, harmony and vitality occurs when Spiritual Ego facilitates the synchronization of the frequencies of our bio-energetic self with the natural rhythms of the Universe
- When we 'sense into self and other' energetically at soul level the resonance of pattern interference will disclose common themes and areas of misalignment

Science of Active Receptivity

A nurse-healer in the postmodern world creates an atmosphere of openness and safety which invites candor, clarity and truth to enter. The maturing Spiritual Ego of the nurse resonates with attributes such as compassion, respect and honesty. This nonjudging, honoring presence is recognized by the Soul of the other person, irrespective of their level of consciousness, creating a felling of safety. In this state of harmlessness, the Soul of the person who has been disrupted by the illness event steps forward to be heard. For some, it is their first encounter with this deeper aspect of themselves. This shared spiritual environment potentiates the self-healing capacity of both the person and the nurse.

The *physical aura* is a vibration of Vital Body cells that create an electrical-chemical movement which forms a light aura around the body; radiating the 'Essence of the Body'. Some healing practitioners can visualize this field as an indicator of physical health. The movement of brain cells create brain waves and the *mental aura*; radiating the 'Essence of Thought'. While EEG readings measure the electrochemical patterns of the brain, mental clarity and emotional state also reflect the health of the mental aura. And, finally, we emit a *quality aura*—Presence—radiating as the 'Essence of Being'. This magnetic field environment radiates from our outer heart chakra; the Soul. It reflects our Spiritual Ego just as the personality is a reflection of our body-mind ego. Although it cannot be observed, it can be felt as an 'atmosphere' much as the climactic conditions of the earth (Fisher, 1996, pp. 93–103).

The Spiritual Ego, which reflects the maturity level of our Soul, is comprised of three levels:

- *Will* is the intent behind the creative impulse. When put forward with resolve—will power—it calls forth a germinal idea and begins the process of movement toward form.
- *Wisdom* is the intelligence of the Soul—Inner Wisdom. As the soul continues to develop, wisdom becomes increasingly inspired by love and expressed under the guidance of will and pure intent. It is vastly greater than anything that can be expressed by the mind. People with a well-developed soul can 'read' the Akashi Records which hold the universal record of all events across time.
- *Love* is the intelligence of the Universe. The highest level of vibration in the Universe, it connects the soul to Universal Wisdom and creates a sense of Unity and Oneness with All-That-Is. Not an emotional feeling, love is the essence of the Universe. It flows into the Soul in increasing amounts as the vibratory capacity of the person expands.

Our Spiritual Ego facilitates a sense of balance and harmony, enhancing vibration as we naturally synchronize the frequencies of our bioenergetic self with the rhythms of the Universe. Soul-facilitated thought fosters responsive rather than reactive decisions, right timing and full utilization of all our potential. From a centered position we see clearly the reality in front of us. We can sense into ourselves and into others, identifying common themes and areas of mis-alignment. As we align with our destiny, synchronicity (which is always present) is increasingly recognized and incorporated into our lives. Living in harmony with the Universal flow, our vibrational resonance draws needed information, resources, and opportunities to us in life-enhancing ways.

The center for the 'Essence of the Divine', our Spirit—our unique spark of life from the Source—is located in the Causal Body which wraps around the entire bioenergetic human energy field, offering protection and access to Divine Universal Consciousness. Our bioenergetic body takes up a unique space in the Universe; it is a node on the Universal Matrix. Energy emitted from our Causal Body is experienced by All-That-Is through the interference pattern created by our vibrational resonance. From this connection, in a moment of total stillness, as in deep meditation, we have access to all Universal Wisdom.

Within the Spirit of humanity reside Universal Spiritual Qualities which are common to all. The best of being human resides within each of us, waiting to potentiate within our Soul as our spiritual/vibrational capacity increases. The Focal Point begins to reside in Higher Mind, allowing the Spiritual Ego to dominate our life, with the personality assisting rather than controlling thought. Body/Mind/Spirit becomes our way of being in the world, and the Universal Qualities increasingly become realized (Price, 1997, pp. 51–59).

Evolution of the Soul—Our Life's Purpose

> *Love inspires Wisdom*
> *Wisdom directs Will*
> *Will controls Active Intelligence*
> *Active Intelligence expresses will, wisdom, & love equally*
> *This is the path of dynamic balance*

Spiritual qualities cannot be learned, they simply are, as manifest in babies and small children. Across the life span we are always capable of experiencing and expressing love, joy, courage, trust, and so on. However, as we begin to mature, logic and control increasingly take over our lives. The spontaneous expression of these qualities gets covered by learned behaviors and self-control. Much as a fish is unaware of water unless placed on dry land, we cannot identify with these qualities as they are within us. To re-member them we must simply be in touch with them. And this requires surfing between the regions of analytic and abstract thought, which is initiated through the expression of 'slow feelings'.

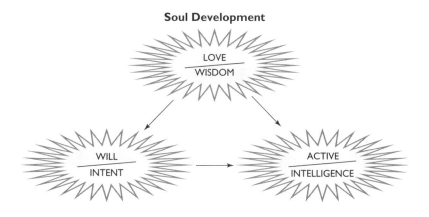

Emotions are always present at the body-mind level, playing a very important part in human evolution. Before joy there was fear; without fear there can be no survival. Brain research has demonstrated that 'fast feelings' of fear and aggression belong to the reptilian and mammalian brain as part of the survival instinct (Lipton, 2005). Stimulated by emotions felt at the body level, they are reactive in nature, creating an immediate response in our concrete world. As we continue to develop associations between real and perceived 'threats' our body-mind cannot discern between doing and thinking about doing. This creates a hindrance not only for the manifestation of our qualities, but also for the manifestation of 'slow feelings', the vehicle in which the spiritual qualities are carried. (Figure 4.4)

The neocortex and our newly forming forebrain (an evolutionary emergence) are home to higher mental functions; abstract thought, planning, complex memories, language, executive reasoning, and the autobiographical sense of self. 'Slow feelings', such as inner peace, stillness, compassion, love, and joy, are not necessary for survival, but are essential to foster the continued unfolding of human potential. Entirely structured in the neocortex, forebrain, and the heart energy vortex, they create 'out-of-body consciousnesses'. Awareness coming from this place creates an atmosphere of nonaction, an environment of stillness.

Real 'power' is simply the awareness to create our own reality, to live our own life and fulfill our destiny. This occurs when we effectively manage both 'fast' and 'slow' feelings. Dynamic balance occurs when we can catch our 'fast feelings' and shift

FIGURE 4.4

Mind-Body-Spirit Model

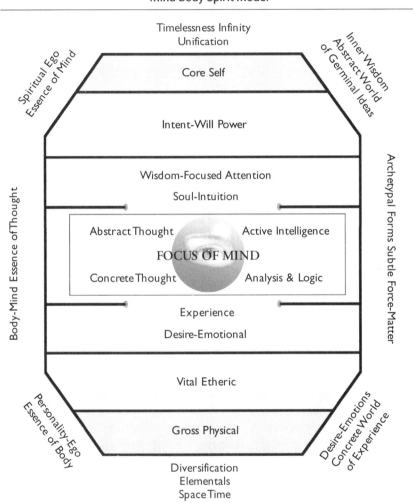

SOURCE: Adapted from B.S. Fisher (1996), *Man, grand reflections of greater cosmic studies in occult anatomy* (Vol. 3) (Prescott, AZ: Sugru Publications), p. 15.

that energy to our higher abstract world guided by 'slow feelings'. Catching a thought creates a huge shift in perception as we experience a break with programmed response; a tiny moment of silence. Stillness is the underlying consciousness out of which every thought-form is born. Wisdom comes with the ability to be still. Being still, looking, and listening activate the nonconceptual intelligence within us, which then directs our words and actions. It also fosters self-healing.

Each health challenge is a manifestation of the body's quest for wholeness (Schoch, 2005, p. 141). Whether we are the nurse or the other person, we must be able to witness the chaos in the illness event so that we can facilitate the reconnection process. This requires the courage of presence. To be totally present, to just observe with awareness, means we must make a relationship with the phenomenon, an act of unconditional love. Thinking and understanding limit the flow of love, while respect and unconditional regard guarantee more consciousness.

When the Soul experiences the presence of total acceptance from another—or from oneself—it encounters real respite, often for the first time. Suddenly, we see the truth that 'weaknesses' are not so much the product of ourselves as they are part of being human. It is the dawning of a deep understanding that these same fears and phenomenon are present in every human being in differing situations and conditions. The structure of life's challenges comes out of the nature of being human, complete with the challenges, fears and emotions that living creates. It is a natural phenomenon, rather than a fatal personal flaw. This realization moves us closer to creating a relationship with ourselves, often for the first time. Things begin to fall into place; the journey toward wholeness has begun.

The doorway to self-healing is sadness. Sadness exists when we become aware that there is no way of doing, no way of achieving, no way of any possible action, not even through fear or anger to change the current situation. Then there is only sadness which stops us in our tracks. This sudden 'not doing' creates a profound stillness; sadness is stillness. Through depersonalization, sadness is immediately transformed into stillness. When we feel self-compassion and surrender, rather than self-pity and struggle, stillness will emerge. Stillness turns into a breathtaking emptiness, not devoid, but filled with totality. Energy not directed toward anything. This energy, full but not used, is compassion; a sense of compassion for ourselves. It activates the Spiritual Ego, and inner wisdom guides action toward a different response. Rather than logic or control, movement flows forward on the energy of love . . . love in action.

Sadness, generated by the realization that our history has ended, moves us from fear and struggle to the acknowledgment of the hopelessness of the situation—and we surrender. The moment of surrender unleashes a sudden feeling of strength. It creates a deep space of stillness and awareness, generating a feeling of closeness. Surrender marks our self-initiated launch on a deeply healing journey. We effortlessly begin to observe what is there. We quit asking why, we do not analyze it; we simply step outside of time into the moment. We let whatever comes up to touch us.

Nurses can help patients move from sadness, to silence, and then forward to healing. Crossing the bridge of sadness moves through several stages (Schoch, p. 155):

- *Learning to Release*—Practicing forgiveness
- *Learning to Be Aware*—Moving into stillness
- *Being in Relationship*—Connecting with things and people meaningful in our life
- *Having Inner Peace*—Having no need for justification
- *Having No Reaction*—Reacting with 'slow feelings' through balanced thought
- *Being Humble*—Having no need for defending; trusting in the Universe

The turning point in an illness event occurs when we no longer feel a need to blame a person or event, make excuses for ourselves, or deny the truth of the situation. The less defensive we are the more love we experience. It is the moment of true surrender; a beginning of trust in the Universe. The attitude of not defending activates the soul. The soul is the only thing worth protecting, and paradoxically, it is protected best by not defending. Simple, loving and compassionate presence-to-self offers a field of total acceptance so there is no need to defend. Self-healing then begins.

Putting it All Together

Traditional nursing practice utilized the scientific process of assessment, diagnosis and intervention and evaluation. The relational paradigm utilizes the process of pattern recognition; exchanging, communicating, relating, valuing, choosing, moving, perceiving, feeling and knowing (Madrid & Barrett, 1994; Newman, 1986; Parse,

1995; Watson, 1999). Inductive clustering of information coupled with deductive selection of crucial concepts guides the nurse's clinical reasoning process (Pesuit & Hermann, 1999). Blending the art, science and presence of nursing into an integrated practice provides access to, and information about the entire bioenergetic system of those we serve. This approach facilitates the self-healing capacity of both the person and the nurse.

Postmodern Nursing: Art/Science/Presence

Contemporary Nursing Practice	Transpersonal Nursing Presence
Scientist and Artist	Witness and Presence
(Logical Analytic Function)	(Active Perceptive Function)
Clinical Competence: Doing For	Compassionate Care: Being With

Nursing Process		
• Current Situation	Assessment	• Larger Context
• Data and Information	Analysis	• Personal/Life Patterns
• Needs and Resources	Planning	• Importance/Meaning
• EBP Plan of Care	Implementation	• Cocreate Unique Response
• Benchmark to Standards	Evaluation	• Growth in In-Sight— Healing

The traditional steps to the nursing process in the clinical domain are matched by a similar inquiry in the spiritual realm.

- *Assessment* includes both the current situation as well as relevant issues in the larger context of their life—as defined by the person
- *Analysis* uses logic to create information out of data while person/family stories and observations over time reveal patterns within the person and the situation at hand
- *Planning* focuses on clinical needs and material resources needed while perception notes the person's actions and reactions energetically, sensing what has greatest importance/ meaning to them so issues are prioritized appropriately
- *Implementation* incorporates the best of standards and evidence based practice that is in accord with patient wishes/ needs/beliefs/expectations, while helping them include things intangible and unique that speak to their deeper needs and wishes

● *Evaluation* involves clinical benchmarks that identify the physiological and psychological advances; while the person's own sense of insight, resolution, or resignation with peace indicate the of level of healing that has occurred soul-wise

When information and perception are considered together in an authentic nurse-person relationship, compassionate care is provided in a relevant way.

BECOMING A HEALING PRESENCE

There is nothing in this world that does not involve a movement toward the soul. Nursing is a practice of serving. It has two aspects; one is to serve others, and the second, deeper meaning is the recognition that our whole being is in the service of our Soul. Our presence can facilitate or hinder others in their healing efforts. Only in transpersonal relationship can each become the carrier of healing energy and love, facilitating the movement toward self-healing and wholeness of both in their own unique way.

Each soul has its pattern of energy, its fundamental evolutionary movement, which means it has a clear purpose—a reason for being—which is to become what it holds within itself. Soul growth is the movement of becoming, not in the sense of knowledge or achievement, but as a blossoming into that which is dormant within us, similar to the unfolding of a flower. As our 'being' deepens we manifest a body that can touch and be touched by others. It has looseness and a translucent quality of radiance about it. This creates an atmosphere where our innate spiritual qualities and our unique personal potential come together into a unified state of being.

The wider the gap of silence between perception and thought, the more depth there is in our being; the more conscious we are. It is this rhythm between doing and being, 'thinking and allowing' which creates the unique characteristics of one's atmosphere; it is the atmosphere of the whole that is important. Spiritual qualities are shared by all of humankind. These are the universal qualities that connect us as One. The more we cultivate them into consciousness, the more they radiate from our essence, inviting those same qualities to surface in another. Qualities that facilitate a healing presence include (Schoch, p. 219):

- *Awareness*: Enlarging perspective which grows out of observation coupled with releasing old patterns and a growing sense of detachment: The stance of witness
- *Respect*: Seeing things as they are by not adding or taking away, coupled with no desire to manipulate or change them
- *Acknowledgment*: Saying 'yes' to an observation without judgment; affirming whatever we see, 'it is what it is'
- *Gratitude*: Recognizing life and its qualities, nothing more than that
- *Humility*: Refraining from power games and egoism, a stance of 'being' that reaches beyond arrogance or struggle. Humility creates protection for the soul in the world.
- *Simplicity*: Allowing what is there to be without adding anything that does not belong; not to lie or betray or exaggerate
- *Trust*: Practicing the art of patience while not being concerned about time; trust can only come through when in the atmosphere of congruence where truth will prevail
- *Surrender*: Forgetting ourselves; it is faith in a process larger than ourselves
- *Vulnerability*: Allowing ourselves to be open to hurt in the psychospiritual sense, which creates strength
- *Love*: Moving toward what is new, which is following the flow of love; embracing and honoring the growth and change in all things

Each unique soul has a blend of characteristics that can be sensed as they are manifest in the actions and attitudes of the individual. If we live in dynamic balance between the analytic and abstract world, we 'walk in balance' within an atmosphere of harmlessness. We are not going anywhere—not into the past or the future; there is only the moment. There is no stability either because there is only change. It is in this atmosphere that one becomes free so the soul can fly.

From this stance we learn to trust our observations without making a single compromise because of what other people say. It is our own observations, made from a heightened state of awareness that can transform us. True presence takes courage and authenticity, which means we must stay with our observations even if they look totally wrong. Our own observations are better and closer to the/ our truth. Resulting decisions and actions are in keeping with the natural 'flow' of the situation before us and the Universe at large.

In order to understand and express ourselves we need a certain amount of space. Providing a space for reflection and contemplation is a key requisite to healing. The less a nurse is in touch with their own atmosphere, the less space they can give the patient. When we are in the presence of suffering, if we constantly try to find ways to help, it will disturb the process of the person's crossing over the bridge of sadness. As a professional caregiver, attachment to our techniques and protocols must be loose enough to allow what is new and unknown to shine through. Practices that support, rather than deny, the suffering of those we serve includes the cultivation of the still point of the heart (Tolle, 2005):

- *Cultivate Stillness*: To be in stillness means being in total insecurity with no reaction, no knowing and no expectation.
- *Cultivate No-Thought*: Observation is the absence of thought that wants to achieve, to change, to 'avoid insecurity'.
- *Cultivate Emptiness*: To be in emptiness means to be content with the 'is-ness' of the moment. Stillness and emptiness, in movement together, becomes the vehicle for manifestation of our soul qualities.

A healing presence is the manifestation of unconditional acceptance. Transpersonal caring is a loving movement out of stillness, the movement toward integration of body, mind and Spirit. In sharing, the unfolding of soul begins. Sharing is the ultimate movement . . . and only a world of sharing is truly a peaceful world.

Living from the perspective of Spiritual Ego versus. personality ego is not something we create. There is nothing special going on. "I am awake," becomes a state of being, only experienced by an outside source. We will not be aware of how loving we are, but others will experience our love toward them. Qualities are manifest only when we are not aware of them, when we have BECOME the qualities . . . when we ARE the atmosphere. Awareness is the absence of description; it is flow. The body-mind stops 'doing and thinking' and becomes instead, a carrier of energy and the qualities, much as a candle hosts the qualities of the flame. Our healing presence becomes the light for others on our shared journey toward wholeness.

> Every illness is a desperate search of the body-mind to again be in relationship with its soul—to regain the ability to radiate the light of love. Consciousness is created through love; a phenomenon of 'knowing' that transcends understanding. When we try to understand something intellectually we limit the movement of the vibrational energy of love which is unconditional and unlimited. The key to healing is total awareness; not just acceptance of what is in front of us, but a direct observation of whatever is present and the process that is unfolding. As the mind quits trying to judge or justify, it begins to relax and quietly observe. Events begin to effortlessly fall into place in a natural rhythm as things become simply what they are intended to be. And we move further down the healing path towards wholeness.
>
> *Manuel Schoch*

Applying the Concepts in Nursing

In order to understand and express ourselves we need a certain amount of space. Providing a space for reflection and contemplation is a key requisite to healing. The less a nurse is in touch with their own atmosphere, the less space they can give the patient. When we are in the presence of suffering, if we constantly try to find ways to help, it will disturb the process of the person's crossing over the bridge of sadness. As a professional caregiver, attachment to our techniques and protocols must be loose enough to allow what is new and unknown to shine through. "Practices that support, rather than deny, the suffering of those we serve includes the cultivation of the still point of the heart" (Tolle, 2005).

Checking In

Cultivation of Relationship from the Still Point—an Exercise.

A healing presence is the manifestation of unconditional acceptance. Compassionate caring is a *movement out of stillness*, the movement toward seeing the other; body, mind and soul. In stillness, the unfolding of soul begins. How comfortable are you with stillness? What practices are you engaged in that cultivate the Still Point within yourself?

Review the following attributes and answer the questions below:

- *Cultivate Stillness*: To be in stillness means being in total insecurity with no reaction, no knowing and no expectation. Question—How comfortable are you with silence?
- *Cultivate No-Thought*: Observation is the absence of thought that wants to achieve, to change, to 'avoid insecurity.' Question—How comfortable are you with change?
- *Cultivate Emptiness*: To be in emptiness means to be content with the 'is-ness' of the moment. Stillness and emptiness, in movement together, becomes the vehicle for manifestation of our soul qualities.
  Question—How comfortable are you without structure?

Reflect on a patient encounter that was particularly meaningful to you, and remember the following:

- What did I communicate to the person when I was with them that was meaningful?
- What did I notice or feel in the exchange that indicated to me that it was particularly important or meaningful to them?
- What gift did I receive from the person in this reciprocal relationship?
- How quiet was the chatter in my mind during our encounter?
- What did the person reflect back to me that gave me an indication of what they were experiencing from me during the exchange?
- Did I have any expectation of rewards from supporting the person?
- What personal growth did I gain from supporting someone, and what would I do differently next time?

Focusing on the relationship rather than the technique creates quality in the exchange. A mutual relationship offers the opportunity for both to grow.

A Living Example

Because it is the human condition to be in relationship with others, we are in a constant state of service. We serve others simply by existing. We serve even when we are not conscious of serving.

I was on a train going through Europe on a cold and rainy day. The train was slowing down to pull into the station. For some reason I became intent on watching the raindrops on the window. Two separate drops, pushed by the driving wind, merged into one for a moment and then divided again-each carrying with it a part of the other. Simply by that momentary touching, neither was what it had been before. And as each one went on to touch other raindrops, it shared not only itself, but what it had gleaned from the other. I saw that metaphor many years ago and it is one of my most vivid memories. I realized then that we never touch people so lightly that we do not leave a trace. Out state of being matters to those around us, so we need to become conscious of what we unconsciously share so we can learn to share with intention (Trout, 1990, p. 254).

Web Site Resource: Sometimes a Healing Presence never disappears. Think of loved ones who have transitioned. Remember the nurse who practiced this principle before it was popular thought. Capture multiple perspectives on this amazing heroine of nursing at *http://www.answers.com/topic/florence-nightingale*

BIBLIOGRAPHY

Bohm, D. (1981). The physicist and the mystic—is a dialogue between them possible? A conversation between David Bohm and Renee Weber. *Re-Vision, 6*(1), 34–44.

Braud, W. (2000). Wellness implications of retroactive intentional influence: Exploring an outrageous hypothesis. *Alternative Therapies, 6*(1), 37–48.

Castenada, Carlos. (1972). *Journey to Ixt.* Carlsbad, CA: Hay House.

Djwal Kul, K. (1996). *The human aura: How to activate and energize your aura and chakras.* Corwin Springs, MT: Summit University Press.

Dossey, B., Keegan, L., Guzetta, C. R., Kolkmeier, L. G. (1995). *Holistic nursing: A handbook for practice* (2nd ed.). Gaithersburg, MD: Aspen Publishing Company.

Dwyer, W. W. (2004). *The power of intention: Learning to co-create your world your way.* Carlsbad, CA: Hay House.

Fisher, B. (1996). *Man grand reflection of the greater cosmos: Studies in occult anatomy* (Vol. 3). Prescott, AZ: Subru Publications.

Hicks, J. (2006). *The amazing power of deliberate intent: Living the art of allowing.* Carlsbad, CA: Hay House.

Hollick, M. (2006). *The science of oneness: A worldview for the twenty-first century.* New York, NY: O Books.

Kuthumi, D. K. (1996). *The human aura.* Corwin Springs, MT: Summit University Press.

Kurtz, E., & Ketcham, K. (1992). *The spirituality of imperfection: Storytelling and the search for meaning.* New York, NY: Bantam Books.

Lipton, B. (2005). *The biology of belief: Unleashing the power of consciousness, matter and miracles.* Santa Rosa, CA: Mountain Love Books.

Madrid, M., Barrett, E. A. M. (Ed.). (1994). *Roger's scientific art of nursing practice.* New York, NY: National League for Nursing Press.

Newman, M. (1986). *Health as expanding consciousness.* St. Louis, MO: C. V. Mosby Company.

Parse, R. R. (1995). *Illuminations: The human becoming theory in practice and research.* New York, NY: National League for Nursing Press.

Pesuit, D., Hermann, J. (1999). *Clinical reasoning: The art & science of critical & creative thinking.* Boston, MA: Delmar Publishers.

Price, J. R. (1997). *A spiritual philosophy for the new world.* Carlsbad, CA: Hay House, Inc.

Rasha. (2003). *Oneness.* Santa Fe, NM: Earthstar Press.

Schoch, M. (2005). *Healing with qualities: The essence of time therapy.* Boulder, CO: Sentinent Publications, LLC.

Tolle, E. (1999). *The power of now: A guide to spiritual enlightenment.* Novato, CA: New World Library.

Tolle, E. (2003). *Stillness speaks.* Novato, CA: New World Library.

Tolle, E. (2005). *A new earth: Awakening to your life's purpose.* New York, NY: Penguin Group USA.

Trout, S. (1990). *To see differently: Personal growth and being of service through attitudinal healing.* Washington, DC: Three Roses Press.

Watson, J. (1999). *Postmodern nursing and beyond.* New York, NY: Churchill Livingston.

Woody, C. (2004). *Standing stark: Willingness to engage.* Prescott, AZ: Kenosis Press.

CHAPTER 5

QUANTUM HEALING
THE POWER OF INTEGRATION

Perhaps each of us has a starved place,
each of us knows deep down what we need to fill that place.
To find the courage to trust and honor the search,
to follow the voice that tells us what we need to do,
even when it doesn't seem to make sense, is a worthy pursuit.

Sue Bender

Illness is part of the human health experience; no one gets through life without some form of physical ailment. Whether it's the common cold, a lingering chronic illness, or life threatening event, every living organism will inevitably encounter a moment when the body is suffering and in need of attention.

What have been your personal experiences with illness? An instructive paradox exists within our profession; at times we are the nurse and at other times the person who is ill. Whether it is ourselves personally or a family member or loved one, we each encounter illness at some point in our lives. It is important to reflect on the lessons learned and attitudes assumed, for, just like those we serve, we come to the healing experience with a set of beliefs and expectations that color the exchange in interesting ways!

HEALTH BELIEFS—LIVING OUR DEFINITIONS

How do you define health—and illness? Our beliefs and definitions guide our nursing practice. If health is the absence of disease, we approach the patient with an arsenal of weapons to conquer the body invaders in warrior fashion. If, on the other hand, it is about balance in multiple dimensions of being, the approach seeks to restore what is innately within and around the individual being supported. Becoming clear about our own health beliefs is the first step to actualizing our professional accountability to others.

Newton's linear and dualistic world views health as the absence of disease. This pervading world view treats health as a commodity that we can acquire if perfect self-control is maintained. We tend to judge those who are considered less diligent in their health practices, including ourselves. In such a world "war" is waged on things that threaten the body. Like the "surgical bombing" carried out in the Iraq War, we attack the invader with antibiotics to kill it, surgery to remove it, or radiation to destroy it.

There is decided value of "good" for health, whereas illness is seen as "bad" and undesirable. Healing practices are prescribed. The healer "knows" what is best, labeling the patient "noncompliant" if orders are not obeyed. This model of practice has been carried out for hundreds of years. However, a new paradigm for health is emerging, one asserting that *disease is a manifestation of health* (Newman, 1986).

The Theory of Complementarity states that two opposites, in relationship, create a whole. Quantum physicist David Bohm observed (Bohm, 1980, p. 39):

> When you trace a particular absolute notion to what appears to be its logical conclusion, you find it to be identical with its opposite, and therefore the whole dualism collapses. Reason first shows you that opposites pass into each other, and then you discover that one opposite reflects the other, and finally, you find that they are identical to each other—not really different at all.

Our journey across the lifespan is a movement toward authenticity, peace, and community. As nurse theorist Margaret Newman helped her mother navigate through a terminal illness, she noticed something intriguing; the more debilitated her mother became, the more she experienced wholeness and peace. Years later that observation matured into her theory called *"Health as Expanding Consciousness"*: Health is an ever-increasing awareness of ourselves and who we are in relation to life in all its fullness, an unfolding of our essence and our destiny (Newman, 1986, p. 37).

Newman believes that health is the expansion of consciousness that transcends the illness–wellness dichotomy. She notes that illness fosters a chaotic energy breakdown, which allows for integration and movement toward new order. The nurse assists with pattern recognition, and through a therapeutic but nonintervention focused relationship, assists the person in gaining new awareness that facilitates an enlarged perspective on life.

Another nursing theorist, Dr. Martha Rogers, also surpassed the prevailing dualistic view between health and disease in her conceptualization of unitary being. Her work asserts that being and becoming, spirit and matter, in fact all dualities, are artificial dichotomies. Rogers views the world as a single unitary energy field that generates, supports, and evolves. In her nonlinear world, things are defined as circular, cyclical, and rhythmical, with relationship central; in relationship we "become manifest" (whether with another person, with the environment, or with one's own higher self). She encouraged nurses to take their practice focus from procedural tasks and physical body symptoms to the higher realm of independent, health-promoting, noninvasive energy-based therapeutic systems. As part of the rhythmic world process of higher frequency, the healer offers a compassionate, nonjudgmental, conscious presence that potentiates the field for the other person's own self-healing (Rogers, 1970).

In each model, health, which encompasses both disease and nondisease, can be regarded as the explication of the underlying pattern of the person environment. This shifting paradigm invites us to expand our viewpoint from looking at parts to looking at patterns. The pattern is information that depicts the whole, understanding the meaning of all the relationships at once. It is a fundamental attribute of the Universal Field, giving unity to the rich diversity within it (Capra, 1988, p. 17).

It is the pattern of our lives that identifies us, not the things that go into making up the pattern. Pattern is relatedness, which includes movement, diversity and rhythm, and energy fields of light and sound. This process is intimately involved in both energy exchange and change or transformation, for as energy is exchanged, the relationships within that pattern are altered (Young, 1976).

Within the past 40 years, the acquisition of knowledge and information has accelerated at a pace beyond that seen on this planet in all of recorded history. New information systems and the widespread access of books have given us an unprecedented, accumulated wealth of knowledge. Through the process of triangulation, we can view a phenomenon of health through physical, psychosocial, and spiritual dimensions, giving an expanded view of reality. When assessed through the lens of Active Intelligence, intuition (which is the subtle art of pattern recognition) adds a deeper understanding to the observation made by logic. This converts data and information to knowledge, which is the foundation for clinical reasoning, the hallmark of a reflective professional nurse.

Noted physician Larry Dossey has identified three eras that provide a framework for the medicine operational in the Western world today. The 1860s ushered in Era I, as science was incorporated into medical practice. During this period, the prevailing assumption was that health and illness were completely physical in nature, with a person's consciousness a by-product of the chemical, anatomic, and physiological aspects of the brain.

Era II emerged in the 1950s with therapies reflecting a growing awareness that a person's mind consciousness, which includes thoughts, emotions, beliefs, attitudes, and meaning, exerts an impact on the body. From this perspective, consciousness was viewed as a "local" phenomenon within the body and in the present moment of a single lifetime.

Era III, the newest and most advanced, is nested within the quantum physics paradigm. Here consciousness is seen as nonlocal and not bound to one individual body. In this world, the minds of humankind are spread throughout space and time. They are infinite, immortal, omnipresent, and ultimately, one. In this space, a person can raise themselves above the day-to-day routines to experience a "transpersonal" experience outside of the local self (Dossey, 1982). As Dossey's rich research demonstrates, healing is affected by building bridges of consciousness with intercessory prayer, certain emotions (i.e., love, compassion), shamanic healing, and miracles. His observation is as follows (1993, p. 86):

> We have nothing to lose by a reexamination of fundamental assumptions of our models of health; on the contrary, we face the extraordinary possibility of fashioning a system that emphasizes life instead of death, and unity and oneness instead of fragmentation, darkness and isolation.

In this era, we are invited to become aware, each moment, of our inner and outer experiences, of our thoughts and assumptions, and their impact on our world. The therapeutic potential of the mind becomes increasingly clear, fostering a "knowing" that all therapies and all people contain a transcendent quality that cultivates healing. In this space, we cocreate and share the healing experience.

Traditional allopathic methods of healing treat the immediate situation with interventions that manage the symptoms, without eradicating the root cause of suffering. As we come to understand the beautiful and dynamic body as a quantum entity, a nested hierarchy of varying levels of energy and consciousness, a new way of engaging with illness emerges. In this world, we do not have to delve into the past to unearth the origins of our neurosis or traumas. We do not have to resort to distraction as an escape by filling our lives with endless activities or cultivate a "positive mental attitude" to drive out undesirable elements in our behavior. There is nothing to acquire; we have all we need within us.

In this rich multidimensional world, we can choose to treat the "whole person," which includes the physical, emotional, mental, and spiritual aspects of our life, by inviting in the power of soul. The essence of soul consciousness influences the brain via the mind and touches all aspects of the person's nature. In this approach to healing, we invite symptoms and suffering into our space as our guide. We sit with sadness as it slowly offers the rich information that was ignored or suppressed for so long. We work with energy going into and out of the physical body as it navigates through the various levels of energy consciousness. And, we recover the authentic qualities of the soul that were our birthright, fostering integration at the deepest levels. In short, we become whole.

THE HEALING PROCESS—REESTABLISHING FLOW

The feeling of wonder begins with our own body. The closest that nature, others, and existence itself comes to us is through our own miraculous body, which holds the water of oceans, the fire of sun and stars, and the air; our body is a gift from the earth (Osho, 2003). Mind is the inner unseen part of the body, while the body is an external manifestation of the mind; the body is the portal of the mind. The conscious mind comprises only 10% of our reality, while deeper truth is experienced in the loving communion between body-mind. When we relax into the flow of life, we are guided by the gentle and subtle promptings of our "Inner Wisdom" (the 90% of consciousness that lies below the level of normal awareness).

Respect and harmony between body and mind manifest as vibrant health and vitality.

However, we are not the body; we are a conscious awareness that takes up residence in this concrete material form. We are a resident in the body temple, a communal gathering place created from the blending of earth (our body) and sky (our consciousness). When we have a healthy relationship with our spirit, who is a witness observer to our body-mind, we are aware of its needs and honor them. We are conscious of the language we use in speaking to and about our body. By honoring its needs and promptings, we develop a deep trust in our inner wisdom, and a right alignment with the energetic flow of life occurs. If we ignore or marginalize symptoms, they will intensify as the body honors our focus, often at its own peril.

All disease is a result of disharmony between the body (form), the Vital Life Force (energy), and our thoughts (mind). The root cause of all illness is the inhibition of the flow of this Force from the Universal Field, the Source. Most of the blockage occurs in the vital etheric body and the emotional body, with a lesser amount of illness coming from the mental body. True healing occurs when the obstruction to the energy flow is removed. Many physical problems are the result of overstressing the body by forcing it to respond to the more subtle and subjective vibrations of our emotional world. This is where the mass consciousness of the majority of present humanity resides. Some physical conditions emerge from the disharmony acquired in connecting with the collective psyche of humankind.

Illness or damage to the physical body primarily comes from trauma or invasion by an external organism. Illnesses rooted in the vital etheric body manifest as congestion and inflammation between the vital and physical bodies, clogging the energy circulatory pathways in the etheric web. Diseases emanating from the emotional body primarily affect the autoimmune system and the central nervous system. Those arising from the mental body emerge from erroneous or negative thinking, generating destructive thought forms. These forms act directly on the emotional body, crystalizing negative emotions and producing one of the most potent causes of bodily enervation (Fisher, 1996, pp. 75–78). Irrespective of its origin, it will result in either depletion or over-stimulation of energy, affecting the nervous system or key endocrine glands. Unchecked, illness or death will ensue.

Wanigi Waci, Lakota spiritual healer, defines health and wellness for his people in the following way (Koerner, 2004):

Each being; the rock people, the winged, feathered or rooted, holds a divine spark of life. When you see the "beauty" in anything—flower, tree, person—you recognize that spark of life in the other. When we live in harmony with all that is, the energy of the universe flows through us all, filling us with all we need in shared fashion. Health is "living in the flow" while disease is "stepping out of flow." There are two ways that we remove ourselves from the streaming energy flow of life. When we think we are above others, our Ego lifts us above the flow. We must then "take it from others," demonstrating characteristics of competition, greed, or theft of some fashion as we take it from others. The second way illness manifests itself is Wego, a weak ego that places itself below others, and then is always looking for a hand out or a hand up. Health is, in the final analysis, right relationship with everything in the world.

Current diagnostic techniques focus on assessment and evaluation of the physical body. However, a comprehensive assessment of illness must include several dimensions beyond the physical symptoms if true healing is to be fostered. Evaluating the primary nature of the cause would include a consideration of factors that are psychic or subjective, inherited or genetic, as well as possible disharmony with the collective human psyche. Methods of treatment would expand beyond conventional allopathic medicine. While it remains a viable and often essential treatment form, others would also be utilized to foster deep healing and integration.

Infusion or redirection of vital energies is enhanced through Ayurveda practices developed in India, Acupuncture and Chinese Medicine, chakra balancing with homeopathy, and psychology. Mind-body medicine addresses issues around emotional and mental imbalance. Hypnosis, biofeedback, guided imagery, psychoanalysis, meditation, yoga, Christian Science, and Faith Healing all assist with slowing down the mind to reconsider the false meaning attributed to an event or issue as well as facilitating management of stress (Goswami, 2004). Play and creativity would foster deepening of the intuition and greater flexibility of mind, increasing insight and resilience. Practices in gratitude and generosity enlarge capacity and connection with the individual and universal soul, aligning us more closely to the flow of universal energy.

Healing is a life-long journey for each of us; it is the human condition. The context for the creation of meaning comes from the consciousness of our Mental-reflective body. Deep healing requires one fundamental action—to take a discontinuous quantum leap in our belief system. The significance we attach to something has a strong influence on its impact to our health (as in the placebo/nocebo affect). Physical illness caused by negative beliefs or memories that impose disharmony on our vital and physical bodies require a change in the meaning context that the mind has established that created the malfunctioning. Physicians Larry Dossey and Deepak Chopra, among others, have identified that rather than drugs or surgery, deep self-healing requires a quantum leap in consciousness (Chopra, 2009):

> Many cures that share mysterious origins—faith healing, spontaneous remissions, and the effective use of placebo, or "dummy drugs"—point toward a quantum leap. Why? Because in all of these instances, the faculty of inner awareness, mediated by the spiritual ego, promotes a drastic jump—a quantum leap—in personal insight—the true mechanism for healing.

This quantum leap is a creative act, coming from the highest level of our consciousness. It is this consciousness of the causal body that has the requisite wisdom (encoded in our spiritual ego), the capacity to discover what is needed (uncovering the life pattern that is the root of the illness), and the power to manifest the insight by unlocking the blocked vital energy at the appropriate chakra, and thus, the physical organ. Our true healing capacity is a self-designed act of ultimate creativity. If we have the courage, energy, and support of others at critical junctures along the way, deep healing occurs as we release old traumas and craft a new perspective on our life.

To foster such a "shift," nurses must partner with the patient as they discern the right path to take rather than "telling them what to do." It is the ultimate misuse of our power to take responsibility for solving problems that belong to others. Our role as witness is to create a safe space for them to sort through the issues of the day, offering understanding and interpretation along the way. Root causes of mental stress include the sense of deep urgency, rush, and hurry, coupled with anxiety and the pursuit of desires for accomplishment. Healing cannot be rushed; illness stops time. A mind that is slowed down is more open and receptive, the first step toward creativity. As we invite patients to stay with their suffering, they become one with it, uncovering the pattern it holds. By inviting them to experiment with various mind-body techniques, using unfamiliar stimuli generates enlarging possibilities by facilitating their *unconscious* processing. Freed from the restraints of mentalization and intellectualism, feelings and vital blueprints become functional once again. Eventually, a seemingly inconsequential trigger precipitates the quantum leap of insight, fostering a release of blocked energy, and true healing begins.

THE HEALING PATH—STAGES OF INTEGRATION

The curing model prevalent in contemporary society can be very beneficial. It offers us comfort in the form of symptom management and time in which to do the more complex work of deeper healing. Oftentimes it can deny rather than facilitate the possibility of healing. The processes used in curing are an attempt to control our experiences, moving them in a prescribed manner and direction toward a predetermined outcome. This approach interferes with our ability to move into unsolicited experiences, the ones required for restructuring our lives. Instead of experiencing the illness event as a step forward toward wholeness, its opposite occurs. However, when used as a stepping stone to multilayered healing, curing can be very constructive.

Healing has little to do with removal of symptoms. Rather, it is an intimate and integrative process that encompasses the entire spectrum of our existence. This daunting journey requires the harmonious alignment of the physical, emotional, mental, and spiritual aspects of our being and how we relate to the world. The outcome of this integration is a greater sense of wholeness and vitality, wellness and soundness, the birthright of every living being (Schoch, 2005).

As quantum physics has demonstrated, a disruptive event offers the space for new order (Levine, 2008). Healing can be viewed as a process of rebuilding one's life anew from chaos and disorder. Psychiatrist Bendit observed (1973, p. 71):

> Healing is basically the result of putting right our wrong relation to our body, to other people....and to our own complicated minds,

with their emotions and instincts at war with one another and not properly understood and accepted by what we call "I" or "me." The process is one of reorganization, reintegration of things which have come apart.

The beginning of the healing journey finds us coming apart at the seams. As we begin to wake up and realize aspects of ourselves we could not previously acknowledge, a deep sadness sets in. By courageously continuing the journey deep into the territory called "The Self," we begin to acknowledge our true condition. Embarking on the task of alignment gives our entire being permission to change in a very natural and automatic way. We initiate the release of old and worn-out thought patterns, and we free blocked emotions and rigid ways of being. We develop a new sense of respect for who we really are, reclaiming the essence of our latent capacities, and the rhythms that are truly ours. Just as a flower opens in the spring, we quietly and naturally unfold and return to our authentic self. Nothing is taken out, nothing is added; we are already whole.

The healing journey moves through predictable stages, leaving in its wake a deep sense of fulfillment, accomplishment, and empowerment (Epstein, 1994). This process is focused on our uniqueness. It involves surrender to both the inner and outer experiences that form our life. It promotes wholeness, allowing the natural rhythms and cycles of our life to be reinstated. It requires forgiveness of others, and offers forgiveness to ourSelf.

Stage I—Embracing our Suffering

Experienced as a different quality from pain, suffering marks the awareness that "something is wrong."

Tenet I of Integrative Healing—Embracing our Suffering

Stage 1- Embracing Our Suffering

The key to healing at this stage is to recognize and surrender to our suffering.

- Begins with physical/emotional pain as symptoms warn that "something is wrong with me."
- Conscious awareness moves beyond pain to suffering—"something is wrong with my life."

(continued)

Tenet I of Integrative Healing—Embracing our Suffering (continued)

- Personality traits or painful childhood memories walled off now surface.
- Patterns for armoring and withdrawing emerge, but we realize "there is no escape here."
- Time stops, and well-intended family, friends, and medical experts tell us what to do.
- Initially we resist suffering through denial, escape, intellectualizing, and distraction.
- TURNING POINT IS SURRENDER, submitting to the suffering.
- Acknowledging the experience, we merge with it, finding its personal theme.
- A breakthrough in awareness shows us our own intuitive world and the wisdom it holds.
- Disconnection from what others tell us to do breaks a barrier in perception.
- Feeling raw and vulnerable, we begin to deal with the deeper issues embedded in the situation.

Role of Practitioner

- Acknowledging their plight gives them confidence and energy to move forward.
- Provide encouragement and support without offering "a solution."

Pain is an awareness of discomfort manifest in symptoms of some fashion. Suffering, however, involves the sense of alienation from our "true self". a recognition that something is wrong, not only with ourselves but also something deep within our lives.

Due to cultural and familial rules and messages, each of us has isolated certain aspects of ourselves, such as personality traits or painful childhood memories, from the rest of our body-mind. Memories of the past freeze our sense of "self" into a rigid and fixed entity, which has been learned in painful events buried in our subconscious history.

In this stage, we are not yet conscious enough to recognize the subtle but profound distinction between our sense of self and our suffering. We think it is all about the illness event. The pain and discomfort of the moment narrows perspective;

a three-dimensional space offers few options for response aside from conditioned patterns of reaction. Our unique pattern for armoring and withdrawing inside of ourselves, learned and activated by painful experiences, emerges as we prepare to bear something from which there is no escape.

Suffering is a natural by-product of a distorted sense of self. Our level of suffering is related to how we perceive the events in our lives. In this stage, we lose touch with normal time–space perception. Time stands still. "Get the doctor" and "What took you so long?" are common comments heard. There is an intensified fear of the future. "What is going to happen to me now?" or "Will this happen again?" are frequent remarks. This stage is very enveloped into the mind; a totally self-focused state of consciousness. There is a felt interference between the core SELF and the way one is living. In essence, an inner voice is crying, "Wake up!" warning us that something is wrong. However, we have ignored that voice for so long that we do not recognize it as our own.

Initially we resist suffering through denial, escape, intellectualizing, or distracting ourselves from direct experience. The constant state of distress is difficult and challenging. The danger is that we can get stuck, spending our entire life in this state of disease. For those with the energy or courage to move forward, the turning point is the simple act of surrender. Growing weary of the struggle, we ultimately stop fighting and begin to work with our suffering. Here a critical shift in consciousness takes place. Roberts has observed (1985, p. 43):

> Here begins the cauterizing, the burning through to the deepest center of being, which is painful and shattering to all aspects of self. The deep deterministic reins of self-control have been taken away and the willpower that glued together this fragile unity has dissolved. From here on, the reins of our destiny are in the hands of a greater power....With no place else to go, nowhere else to turn, we have no choice.

This is an internal spiritual or mental emergency that cannot effectively be treated or cured. Responding to the inner call of distress is all that is required of us. Logic and linear reasoning are no help here. Submitting to the struggle begins our healing.

As others acknowledge our plight, we feel a sense of support, which gives the time and momentum necessary to move forward to the next stage. A simple acknowledgment from family and health professionals is often the energy necessary to begin to move on.

Too often, well-meaning family and friends—and professionals—give advice or opinions about the situation at hand, rather than simply inviting us to engage with our process. A healing presence respectfully witnesses the situation with no judgment or recommendation, allowing us to authentically "show up." As we acknowledge the experience, we empower ourselves to merge with it, resonating with the rhythm of the suffering that lies under the physical or emotional pain. After awhile we become one with it and recognize its theme.

Here an important shift occurs in our consciousness. Suddenly, as if by magic, we sense a subtle change in awareness, sensing a doorway to a new understanding coming from ourSelf. Our total entrapment in consensual reality (a world determined by mass consciousness) breaks open as we catch a glimpse into our own subjective intuitive world and the power and wisdom it holds. Feeling raw, disheveled, and very vulnerable, we sense that a barrier has been broken that kept us confined. This moves us to the second stage.

Stage II- Transcending our Polarities

As we enter this stage, the tendency to judge ourselves and events in our lives intensifies because we now have a "greater sense of I" about ourselves and life around us, rather than scripts from family or mass consciousness.

Tenet II of Integrative Healing—Transcending Our Polarities

Stage II- Transcending Our Polarities

The key to healing at this stage is developing personal awareness and self-responsibility separate from family/mass consciousness.

- Tendency to judge ourselves and events in our lives intensifies as as our insight into ourselves and life around us expands.
- Through projection we place blame outside ourselves, minimizing the power of healing insight.

(continued)

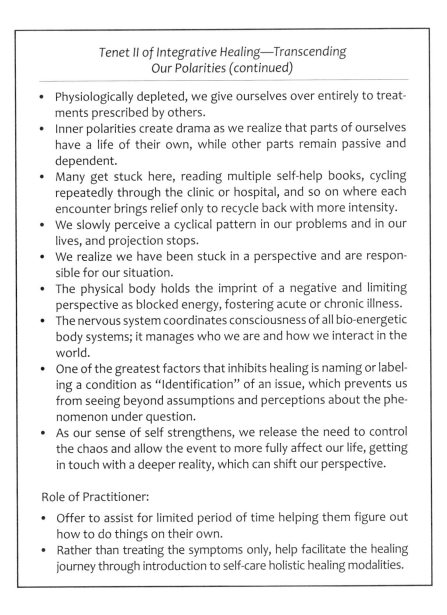

Tenet II of Integrative Healing—Transcending Our Polarities (continued)

- Physiologically depleted, we give ourselves over entirely to treatments prescribed by others.
- Inner polarities create drama as we realize that parts of ourselves have a life of their own, while other parts remain passive and dependent.
- Many get stuck here, reading multiple self-help books, cycling repeatedly through the clinic or hospital, and so on where each encounter brings relief only to recycle back with more intensity.
- We slowly perceive a cyclical pattern in our problems and in our lives, and projection stops.
- We realize we have been stuck in a perspective and are responsible for our situation.
- The physical body holds the imprint of a negative and limiting perspective as blocked energy, fostering acute or chronic illness.
- The nervous system coordinates consciousness of all bio-energetic body systems; it manages who we are and how we interact in the world.
- One of the greatest factors that inhibits healing is naming or labeling a condition as "Identification" of an issue, which prevents us from seeing beyond assumptions and perceptions about the phenomenon under question.
- As our sense of self strengthens, we release the need to control the chaos and allow the event to more fully affect our life, getting in touch with a deeper reality, which can shift our perspective.

Role of Practitioner:

- Offer to assist for limited period of time helping them figure out how to do things on their own.
- Rather than treating the symptoms only, help facilitate the healing journey through introduction to self-care holistic healing modalities.

Phrases such as "a bad back," or "a lousy situation" abound. We also give ourselves over entirely with blind commitment to the procedures and treatments prescribed by others. However, we also begin to notice that there is a polarity within ourselves. Some parts of our being are starting to have a life of their own while others are passive and dependent. Our personality's engagement in judging and evaluating demonstrates that a sense of "me" is developing.

Old patterns of projection often place the "blame" outside ourselves, fostering a danger that may minimize the power of healing insight. Physiologically, we do not have the strength for self-empowerment and so we defer to outside agents easily. Life is experienced as a roller coaster of correcting or being corrected as these newly recognized polarities create drama in our world and relationships.

Many people get "stuck" in this stage of healing. Countless self-help courses, books and diets are consumed by people in this stage. The modern medical establishment and state-of-the-art hospitals are a haven for the cyclical patterns of health-illness in their life. Each encounter, move, or change offers a moment of joy or sense of place, and then, suddenly the pattern repeats. The new job may be worse than the last, the new relationship no more satisfying. The Dalai Lama spoke of this pattern in the dynamic book *Health Through Balance* (1986, p. 37):

> Basically, every being on this planet—wants happiness and does not want any form of disease or suffering. Yet, we do not know how to achieve the causes of happiness and do not know how to get rid of the causes of suffering...We make great efforts at techniques for achieving happiness and avoiding pain, but instead, our efforts mostly generate just the opposite of what we seek—bringing on ourselves more pain and suffering and diminishing whatever happiness we have.

We discover that what we considered hard and fast rules for good and bad, or right and wrong, become muddled as we begin to realize that what we thought was the root of our problem was inaccurate or partial. We slowly begin to perceive a cyclical pattern in our problems and in our lives. We can begin to recognize a certain pattern in our intimate relationships as well as those at work and in the larger world.

While the cycle of each of us is unique, all cycles fit into an underlying form of the natural rhythm of the Universe. From the rise and fall of civilizations to the division of a cell, each cycle fits into the encompassing cadence of earth and cosmos. The Spirit of Universal Consciousness is the timeless wisdom that organizes the universe and also governs the rhythm of our self. Its intelligence resides in our body-mind, guiding us through our own evolution. Disease occurs when we are out of step with our own natural rhythms. Suffering amplifies our natural tendencies, as well as highlighting where the authentic rhythm has been isolated, repressed or denied. As our strict adherence to rigid rules falls away, we begin to connect more deeply with our own natural patterns and awareness grows.

As our insight becomes stronger we quit projecting our problems and ideas onto others, and take them back into ourselves. In this sphere lies the hope for reconciliation of the polarities. We begin to see that instead of life being an endless stream of suffering and drama, it also holds intervals free and open. Our demands, like those of an angry child coming from an unresolved conflict, give way to requests coming from a more healed and integrated awareness. Occasionally we have a sense of déjà vu, recognizing a repeat of something from the past. We start to notice how our judgments manifest in our life, and we begin to identify which of our actions trigger specific responses in others. Victim-minded cause and effect gives way to the recognition that we have a role in the process.

As we develop a stronger sense of self, we acquire the strength to assume greater responsibility for our situation. We realize that we have been stuck in a perspective and that we are responsible for the result. And, we sense that our body is holding the imprint of that belief as blocked energy manifest as an acute or chronic condition. Occasionally we can even place a finger on the location of that "stuck" feeling. However, while we are developing a new body-mind, we still persist in manifesting old patterns. Deepak Chopra observed (1993, p. 79):

> Ninety eight percent of the atoms in our body were not there a year ago. The skeleton that seems so solid was not there a year ago. . . The skin is new every month. You have a new stomach lining every four days, with the actual surface cells that contact food being renewed every 5 minutes. The cells in the liver turn over very slowly, but new atoms still flow through them, like water in a river course, making a new liver every 6 weeks.

As opposed to organs and soft tissue, nerve cells do not regenerate. It is the nervous system that coordinates conscious integration of all body parts, systems and patterns. This powerful mechanism maintains our body's inner environment, acting as a conduit for the expression of Universal Consciousness (our Inner Wisdom). The nervous system manages who we are and how we interact with the world. When it has not been healed from the trauma of past events, our emotional reality is also stuck. Health, well-being, vitality, and wholeness flow from a nervous system that is free of interference.

Life factors that create interference patterns which are disruptive to the flow of consciousness energy include things such as medications, alcohol, environmental pollutants and chemicals in foods, electromagnetic radiation from computers, cell phones and appliances, and airplanes. Physical pressure on the nervous system from trauma, tumors, excessive stretching or twisting and mechanical injury, can also alter the body's ability to heal. Or biography becomes or biology. The combined effects of various stresses and the inability of the nervous system to fully perform its intended functions, leads us to "being stuck." Pierrakos, MD, noted (1987, p. 88):

> The constrictions of energy…are not isolated dysfunctions. They are the blocks of stultified energy that trammel the physical body in skeletomuscular rigidities, and also disrupt the higher planes of energy, thus affecting mental attitudes and expanding consciousness.

Epstein (1994, pp. 48–50) observed that with each position of the spine, there is a corresponding predisposition of consciousness, mood or personality. Being stuck is only partially related to conscious choice, but rather is often a consequence of a fixated nervous system due to a spinal distortion or related problem. Our body movement and tension reveal the history of our physiology, whether we are conscious of it or not.

One of the greatest factors that inhibit healing is the *naming or labeling of a condition*. "You have cancer" gives identification to the issue, but immediately prevents us from seeing beyond the assumptions and perceptions about the phenomenon under question. In nursing, the labels affixed to someone or something, whether in charting, giving a shift report, or conversion with patients, families and coworkers, can be very detrimental to all.

Labels give us shortcuts in communication, but often, they also cut short our exchange with the person or phenomena.

Caring for someone at this stage involves offering to assist for a limited period of time, helping them "figure out what is going on" and how to do things on their own. Such an approach builds a bridge between levels of consciousness that lead to a more expansive perspective. Talking or thinking about a problem does not resolve it, but acknowledging and experiencing it brings it into a personal encounter which can shift perspective. Dr. Lowen wrote (1980, pp. 260–261, 267):

The patient must be brought into touch with reality—the reality of their life situation, the reality of their feelings, and the reality of their body. These three realities cannot be separated from one another. The person who is in touch with their feelings is also in touch with their body situation. By the same logic, the person who is in touch with his body is in touch with all aspects of his life.

Control creates a limited perspective physically, emotionally, mentally and spiritually, contributing to the perpetuation of the current situation. As our sense of self is strengthened, we begin to release efforts to control the chaos, and allow the disruption to more fully impact our life. The more flexible and adaptable we are the easier it is to move through this stage. Individuals who are engaged in exercises such as yoga, aerobics, stretching or athletics move through this stage with a minimum of intervention.

Increasing self-care options by including holistic practices facilitates the healing journey rather than maintaining a curing regimen designed to control symptoms. This stage is facilitated by massage therapy, craniosacral and acupuncture therapies, shiatsu and therapeutic touch practitioners, and nontherapeutic chiropractors. Healing disciplines such as Jungian therapy, bioenergetics, healing touch, Reike, and Rolfing are other venues that can open the person to new ways of connecting with their body mind and moving into the next stage of healing.

Stage III- Moving Toward Authenticity

This stage moves us to reclaiming our personal power while accepting responsibility for our own healing.

Tenet III of Integrative Healing—Moving Toward Authenticity

Stage III- Moving Toward Authenticity

The key to healing at this stage is identifying and merging with the root issues/patterns which keep us from authentic self-expression.

- We reclaim our personal power while taking responsibility for our own healing.
- We start to reject our symptoms and move away from suffering.
- We consider a new direction; change in job or relationship, having surgery.
- Some repeat their old pattern in a new way—new job or marriage—getting tuck in the same old chaos
- At this point relationships are the biggest challenge.
- Rather than deciding what to do, this is a time to reclaim our own truth and wisdom.
- If the path is not yet clear, the body may not be healed enough to accommodate the change.
- When all forms of judgment are removed we can look back without anger or deep emotion, starting to merge with the shadow aspects of our life.
- Releasing the emotional attachment to an event releases blocked energy, infusing us with a sense of emotional, intellectual, and spiritual empowerment and compassion.
- We quit blaming, making excuses or looking for answers; we begin the work of forgiveness.
- A significant nonlocal impact on others also involved in the drama is also made.

Role of Practitioner

- Practitioner moves from authority figure to partner.
- Ask them 'what is the worst thing that can happen?' to help them move beyond fear.

Key phrases include comments such as, "I'm not going to take this anymore!" or "I must honor who I really am." Here we approach the bifurcation point referred to in quantum physics, where the next path is chosen when we make a choice amongst the "strange attractors" inviting us forward (Siegel, 2008).

We begin to reject our symptoms and separate ourselves from our suffering by assuming greater responsibility for the deeper, less obvious facts underlying our situation. Due to our strengthened sense of self, we realize that we have dishonored our inner essence and step out of suffering by moving in a new direction. This may include considering leaving a relationship, undergoing surgery, or quitting a job. The other path, chosen less frequently, involves a sudden and radical quantum leap in consciousness.

Now relationships bring about our greatest challenges because we often attract partners who express the alienated aspects of ourselves. Whatever we repress is often expressed by the partner in an intimate relationship, often around issues of work, finances or relationships. As we reclaim those latent capacities with our-self, it will alter the patterns currently established within existing relationships. This disruption offers everyone an opportunity to create patterns that are in sync with the larger rhythms of their own life, and the dance of the Universe—everyone has a chance to become more whole.

This is not a time to decide what to do, but rather a time to work on reclaiming our own truth and wisdom. When changes are necessary, our Internal Wisdom will always guide us in direction and timing. If the path is not clear, it may be that our body mind hasn't healed enough to accommodate that change. This juncture is the true beginning of the spiritual journey, as noted by Assagioli (1992, pp. 35–38):

> Man's spiritual development is a long and arduous journey, an adventure through strange lands full of surprises, difficulties and even dangers. It involves a drastic transformation of the "normal" elements of the personality, an awakening of the potentialities hitherto dormant, a rising of consciousness to new realms, and a functioning alone in a new inner dimension.

Some will escape the discomfort by producing new versions of the same old patterns in order to control the chaos. "Easy" ways include finding another partner or avoiding relationships altogether. Changing jobs, seeking therapeutic care from some form of practitioner, psychotherapist or financial counselor, are all efforts to regain control in their lives. Many people do not complete this stage of the journey.

Quantum physicists have demonstrated that chaos is an essential aspect of life, a necessary ingredient in the evolutionary process. At the edge of chaos is "the verge" the place of unlimited potential. Bohm has observed (1980, p. 39) that:

> Chaos science uncovers that the irregularities are not devoid of order; that even seemingly chaotic processes such as weather patterns, and turbulence in fluids is found, on detailed analysis, to exhibit subtle strands of order.

Rather than repressing chaos in our lives, when we have the strength to engage with it, inviting chaos into our lives gives us the experience and wisdom of its energy. We then discover the lessons nested in the disruptive event as we uncover the underlying order behind its appearance. As disorder strongly impacts our nervous system, our ability to create order out of chaos is a sign of our growing consciousness.

This stage removes all forms of judgment from our lives. Simultaneously, we make a deeper commitment to wholeness in every aspect of our relationship to our reality. Now we gently take our power with no anger or emotional attachment to pervious events. We can gaze into a photo album, revisiting the place where our suffering began, and gain insight without emotional storms. We have begun the process of merging with our shadow side. It is the beginning of compassion—for others—and for ourSelf.

Here we can observe the process behind our suffering without taking it personally. We look behind the struggle of that event and discover what it has to teach us. We let this process unfold, guided by our Inner Wisdom rather than our educated minds, with profound results. As we release the emotional attachment to the event, it has a significant nonlocal impact on others also involved in the drama.

As we merge with the illusion of past wounds we feel a new sense of empowerment at intellectual, spiritual and emotional levels as well as physically. Blocked energy is released, infusing us with a strength that comes from discovering the "truth," opening us to higher dimensions of consciousness energy. We suddenly realize that suffering is not to be taken personally; rather it is a wake-up call to investigate ourselves and our situation more deeply. *We begin to understand that in therapy we looked for answers and excuses, while in spiritual healing we seek understanding and often, forgiveness.*

At this stage a healthcare practitioner moves from authority figure to becoming a partner. What evolves is a practice partnership, where each is committed to the growth, healing and evolution of the other. Because we are all human, each of us has variations to the theme being played out in the other's life. We each view the central issue from our own stage of development, taking what we need and offering what we have. In this exchange both become more.

The key to healing at this stage is engaging and merging with the issue which fostered the suffering. Resistance to this process occurs as fear of what we imagine may happen overtakes us. As our trusted healing partner asks "What is the worst that can happen?" we can take the next step. Finding out what lay behind the pattern, knowing what we can do differently and how our lives are to change can only be understood when we see clearly without illusion. A trusted associate is invaluable in helping us lay out the issues honestly, then helping guide us to the new perspectives on the other side. Completion of this step takes us to the next stage of healing.

Stage IV- Enhancing Capacity

At this stage we are ready to release aspects of ourselves that cannot adapt to our new and stronger sense of self.

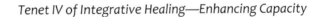

Tenet IV of Integrative Healing—Enhancing Capacity

IV- Enhancing Capacity

The key to healing at this stage is to transcend old blockages and align with natural rhythms of life.

- We are ready to release aspects of self that cannot adapt to new and stronger self.
- Trapped perspectives, memories, energy patterns are released at discretion of our Inner Wisdom.
- This frees up the body-mind to accommodate an enlarging consciousness.
- With increased flexibility and momentum we begin to invite change into our lives.
- Centering and grounding are the assignments at this stage of healing.

(continued)

Tenet IV of Integrative Healing—Enhancing Capacity (continued)

- Lifestyle habits shift as a commitment to wellness practices are made.
- We are drawn to activities that increase aptitude for movement and awareness.
- Discharge of blocked energy occurs only when nervous system is able to accommodate it.
- It is the precursor to integration, experienced as nausea, deep sadness, and emotional anxiety.
- Danger at this stage is that uncomfortable feelings may throw us back to an earlier stage.
- What some perceive as illness is often the body's attempt to discharge or release something to reach a new level of health.
- After discharge a deep resolution occurs, a deep sense of accomplishment, freedom, peace.
- Discharge often includes cleaning out old closets and files, going through wardrobes and relationships; getting one's house in order.

Role of Practitioner:

- It is important to work with a practitioner who can help us move into and through the chaos rather than stopping when it gets uncomfortable.
- Recommend practitioners who foster physical/psychological/emotional centering and grounding .

Trapped perspectives, memories, and energy patterns will be released at the discretion of our Inner Wisdom, freeing up our body-mind to accommodate an enlarging consciousness. With increased flexibility and momentum we begin to invite change into our life. Larry Dossey, MD noted (2001, p. 103):

> Health is harmony, and harmony has no meaning without the fluid movement of interdependent parts. Like a stream that becomes stagnant when it cease to flow, harmony and health turn into disease and death when stasis occurs. We are called to return to the concept of the biodance, the endless streaming of the body-in-flux.

Centering and grounding are the assignments at this stage of healing. We begin to change lifestyle habits, open to new perspectives on healing and commit to wellness practices. Diet and exercise patterns are reviewed. Activities such as meditation, biofeedback and yoga are explored. We naturally gravitate toward activities that increase aptitude for movement and awareness, which enhances our capacity for growth and change. At this stage magical "synchronicity" begins to occur as our body-mind is open and flexible enough to note and accommodate it. Opportunities that align to better our circumstance appear unexpectedly because we are now receptive to them. A danger at this stage is getting preoccupied with the unfolding process. If we become overly concerned or confused, or doubt our Inner Wisdom, we may be thrown back to an earlier stage of healing.

As we move closer toward discharge of a long-held pattern, uncomfortable feelings are manifest. Discharge is the precursor to integration. We must accept that we cannot be healthy unless we go out of control through the process of discharging outmoded ways of knowing and being to accommodate our infinite self. Few people allow their body temperature to rise naturally to 102 to 103 when they are ill. Whenever we interfere with natural body processes, we create more of what our body is trying to eliminate. The discharge will take place when our nervous system is flexible enough to accommodate it.

Symptoms of the discharge process are not a sign of disease, but rather an indication that a healing crisis is moving the body-mind toward resolution and integration. At this point we may experience nausea, deep sadness or emotional anxiety which may foster thoughts of aborting the process. It is imperative that rather than treating the symptoms, we work with a practitioner who can support our further movement into the chaos that is absolutely essential for meaningful change, for lack of needed discharge equals lack of health.

Any aspect of our "self" that no longer works for our best health will be discharged by our innate intelligence. As the Focus Point begins to shift to the higher aspect of body-mind, it will move to eliminate anything, including lifestyle and habits, which no longer serves its highest good. It also discharges the rhythm that cannot live in harmony with the whole. J. Krishnamurti, an Indian philosopher, often taught that to help someone with a problem, all you had to do was understand it without judgment and see it clearly; in time this understanding will be transmitted to the person with the problem. The same holds true for the body.

What many consider as sickness is often the body simply attempting to discharge or release something it does not want in order to reach a new level of health. After the discharge there is a resolution, much as the relief after a sneeze that produces feelings of calm. A deep sense of accomplishment, freedom, and peace is a sign that integration of the dissonance has occurred with higher order, another movement closer to wholeness.

The discharge process also includes cleaning out closets and desks, going through wardrobes and relationships. It literally is a process of "getting one's house in order." We find that we spontaneously release what no longer serves us, making more room and a more flexible system to store material, information and fresh life experiences that are not simply extensions of the past. This all leads to creation of a fuller experience in the present.

Facilitating this movement toward integration requires us to avoid traps which may derail the process. Old patterns in life revisit us in an effort to bring us back including: fear of change, self-resentment which will sabotage the healing process, a personal sense of frustration or deep loneliness, and guilt associated with self-judgment. These feelings prevent us from remaining in the present, drawing us back to earlier stages of our life. Rather than assuming worn out responses, we must remain diligent in maintaining awareness that the process is moving us to the next stage of healing.

Stage V- Emptiness Moving Toward Integration

After discharge is complete, we move toward the moment of emptiness and vulnerability.

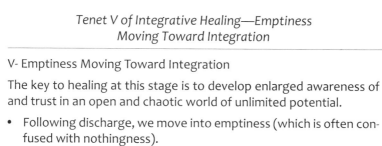

Tenet V of Integrative Healing—Emptiness Moving Toward Integration

V- Emptiness Moving Toward Integration

The key to healing at this stage is to develop enlarged awareness of and trust in an open and chaotic world of unlimited potential.

- Following discharge, we move into emptiness (which is often confused with nothingness).
- We migrate toward a new world of possibilities with a sense of calm, but also aloneness.

(continued)

Tenet V of Integrative Healing—Emptiness
Moving Toward Integration (continued)

- Without common reference patterns of the past, we are unsettled, but aware.
- We start to notice our Higher Self, changing our inner dialogue, sensing connections with ourselves we did not know before.
- The resonance of our newfound awareness begins to attract new objects, people, and experiences into our world.

Role of Practitioner:

- We are now our own practitioner, engaged in self-care activities such as spontaneous expressions of gratitude, prayer, meditation, use of musical instruments as well as our own voice, yoga and T'ai Chi, which all promote integration.

Much as the crab that has outgrown their shell searches for a new home, we move toward a world of new possibilities with a sense of calm, as well as a knowing that in some ways we are alone. This dynamic sets the stage for deeper exploration and movement forward. We feel raw while we also realize that in a silent space we can tune into the sacred within. We are now without our common reference points that have guided us for years. While it opens new room for possibilities, it is also unsettling. Poet Zambucka wrote (1984, p. 58):

> And as you reach new plateaus of thought. . .
>> And old friends drop away,
>> Fear not loneliness,
>> For there is a silent communication between those at the
> same level of awareness.
>> And for the first time you will not be lonely. . . .

Emptiness is often confused with "nothingness," however it is so much more than that. It offers a space for transition from one level of consciousness to another; a place to shift the focal point from the lower mind ego of our personality to our higher spiritual ego (Fisher, 1996, pp. 75–78, 95–99). We experience a sense of freedom as our consciousness is not attached to one particular perspective. In the space of emptiness, the resonance of our newfound awareness will begin to attract objects, people, and experiences into our world. This empty dynamic state of readiness touches the Universal Field. Physicist Talbot notes (1986, p. 156):

> Many physicists believe that at its ultramicroscopic level, empty space is really a turbulent and frothy storm of activity. Moreover. . . within these violent upheavals in the nothingness, new particles are constantly being created and destroyed…..ultimately everything we know as real in the entire universe may originally have sprung out of this empty but seething vacuum.

Thus, all potential realities exist in the field of emptiness, which is a state of "everythingness." Our newfound sense of wholeness and emptiness is a powerful outlook for stepping into the stillness, the place where our own voice can best be heard. We begin to have differing forms of internal dialogue, sensing connections within our-Self that were not present before. There is a danger at this point to move into ascetic practices that deprive ourselves of various things. However, the stronger response is to honor our inner essence and outer experience through aligning with its natural rhythms.

Practices at this stage involve spontaneous expressions of gratitude. Cultivating a deep sense of appreciation for All That Is deepens our connection to the Source. Prayer is another powerful vehicle to express our yearning for relationship and union with the One. Whatever form of religion or spiritual practice one has chosen, "prayer waves" resonate on the subtle realms of existence, building bridges for healing and grace (Dossey, 1993).

The tone of musical instruments and our own voice facilitate deepening the resonance of our body-mind with the universal rhythms and wholeness of spirit. Yogic practices of rhythmic breath and devotion, chanting and singing, or other forms of gentle movement such as T'ai chi, promote integration. Self nurturing practices such as massage, a relaxing hot bath, being held by someone else, are all enjoyable and integrating experiences. As we align more closely with our own rhythm, serendipity is a frequent visitor as we resonate more closely with the rhythms of the universe. New and exciting people come into our lives, people who will uplift us, changing our life in positive ways. As we learn to trust the process, and trust ourselves, a deep sense of peace prevails. Derek Walcott invites us (2001, p. 5):

> The time will come when with elation you will greet yourself,
>> Arriving at your own door, in your own mirror,
>> And each will smile at the other's welcome;
>> Saying, sit here. Eat.
>> You will love again the stranger who was yourself.
>> Give wine, give bread, give back your heart
>> To the stranger who was loved all your life,
>> Whom you abandoned for another, who knows you by heart.
>> Take down the love letters from the bookshelf,
> the photographs,
>> the desperate notes.
>> Sit. Feast on your life.

The mantra of the day becomes simply, "thank you," as you move into the next stage of healing.

Stage VI- Shifting the Focal Point

As we begin to move within this higher state of conscious awareness, we start to perceive that life is more than an outward physical manifestation.

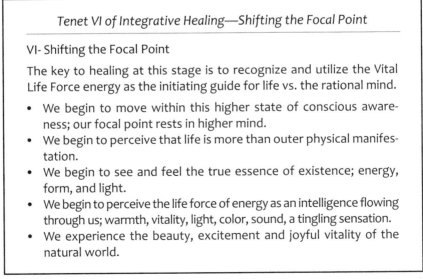

Tenet VI of Integrative Healing—Shifting the Focal Point

VI- Shifting the Focal Point

The key to healing at this stage is to recognize and utilize the Vital Life Force energy as the initiating guide for life vs. the rational mind.

- We begin to move within this higher state of conscious awareness; our focal point rests in higher mind.
- We begin to perceive that life is more than outer physical manifestation.
- We begin to see and feel the true essence of existence; energy, form, and light.
- We begin to perceive the life force of energy as an intelligence flowing through us; warmth, vitality, light, color, sound, a tingling sensation.
- We experience the beauty, excitement and joyful vitality of the natural world.

(continued)

---

*Tenet VI of Integrative Healing—Shifting
the Focal Point (continued)*

- Gratitude and acknowledgments flow from us rather than manipulation and control.
- Thoughts begin to break up from patterned thinking to energy packets of attention.
- We begin to separate from the rest of the world, merging increasingly with the wholeness of our being; feeling safe, connected, and embraced.

We can literally see and feel the true essence of existence; energy, form and the light behind form. We begin to perceive the life force of energy as an intelligence flowing through us. It appears as warmth, vitality, light, color and sound, or a tingling sensation.

For the first time we experience ourselves as part of a larger reality, one comprised of energy rather than physical things. We begin to relate to life beyond physical form, experiencing the beauty, excitement and joyful vitality found in the natural world, and in all things. Redfield provides insight to this phenomenon (1993, p. 17):

> We humans will learn to perceive what was formerly invisible types of energy....Human perception of this energy first begins with a heightened sensitivity to beauty...the perception of beauty is a kind of barometer telling each of us how close we are to actually perceiving this energy.

Gratitude and acknowledgement of the flow of life, as opposed to manipulation and control, are signs that ego investment has been transcended. We do not need to change anything, but rather, be in harmony with the stage we are in, whether for ourselves or others. Epstein has observed that "expecting and honoring what is observed is enough for it to be transformed on its own accord." (1994, pp. 183–186)

At this stage, thoughts begin to break up from patterned thinking to energy packets of attention. Fresh awareness and understanding emerge as we work though the higher intelligence of our spiritual ego, accompanied with feelings of joy, gratitude and love that allow for accommodation of our spirituality and wholeness. Suddenly we are "no one" as our old forms being to dissolve. We begin to separate from the rest of the world, merging increasingly with the unrecognized wholeness of our being. Here we feel safe, connected, embraced and embracing. We are both observing ourselves and experiencing ourselves beyond all boundaries as polarity has been transcended. Paramahansa Yogananda, the beloved teacher of Kriya Yoga, taught that Divine energy flow and connection with the Ultimate One is experienced in eight ways: light, sound, peace, calmness, love, joy, wisdom, and power (Yogananda, 1959). Here there is no sense of separation and everything we touch enriches us. As with every other stage, surrendering fully to the moment empowers us to move to the next stage. However, at this stage compassion is a lens for all we experience (Dossey, 2008).

Stage VII- Returning to Community

We move back into connection with ordinary reality knowing that the source of love and power is enfolded in Universal Consciousness. *It does not come from us, nor does it depend upon us.* This gift from the One is available to all.

Tenet VII of Integrative Healing—Returning to Community

VII- Returning to Community

The key to healing at this stage is to live with timeless awareness in the larger world.

- We move back into connection with ordinary reality knowing that the source of love and power is enfolded in universal consciousness.
- *It does not come from, nor depend, on us.*
- Our expanded world is filled with more energy and a broader perspective.
- We naturally align with life's natural rhythms, uplifting situations around us.
- Our daily practice includes remaining mindful of the miracle of life, and expressing gratitude for its generous gifts.
- We make a commitment to being a deeper healing presence in the world which comes from timeless awareness.

We experience love with no conditions, becoming more open and available to community.

This deep "knowing" transforms the life we continue to live going forward in a more loving and compassionate way. Meditation teacher Jack Kornfield observed (1993, p. 116):

> You have to live your spirituality day to day, at home, at work, in your car. Otherwise, it won't transform you, and in the end you won't benefit and transform the world around you.

Our expanded world is filled with more energy, a broader perspective, and greater understanding. We naturally align with life's natural rhythms, serving as conduits for the universal rhythms, uplifting situations around us as we no longer engage in the drama. Our daily practice includes remaining mindful of the miracle of life, and expressing gratitude for its generous gifts. We make a deeper commitment to being a healing presence in the world. Trungpa observed (1984, p. 85):

> You can invoke and provoke the uplifted energy of basic goodness in your life. You begin to see how you can create basic goodness for yourself and others on the spot, fully and ideally, not only on a philosophical level, but on a concrete physical level.

People and experiences continue to emerge which invite us to liberate ourselves from old perspectives, furthering our growth. We begin to recognize that our thoughts are distractions—concepts, comparisons and analysis are habits which prevent focus on the moment and what is trying to occur. We have come to understand that healing occurs in the moment, which is also the eternal. Dr. Chopra addresses timeless awareness (Chopra, 1993, p. 43):

> Healing comes about through transcendence. There is no other way out. To see things with the crystal clarity of pure awareness not through the old memories, not remaining a victim of the stale repetition of old memories. So we reexperience pain, sorrow, anger, guilt, physical conditions with this new awareness, no longer being attached to them, observing them, observing ourselves, observing the action.

As things are viewed from a larger vantage, we experience love with no conditions. We no longer care if our ideas or offerings are well received; we simply submit them as an authentic gift from the heart. As we become more open and available to others, our sense of community increases.

We begin to see community in everything from the cells that support our body to the cosmic sky. In community, we find places within ourselves where we had lost our participation. We now have healed sufficiently to share our gifts of wisdom, understanding and compassion which were acquired on our healing journey. Sharing our wounds is a sacred act for they contain the seeds of healing for both ourselves and the universe.

Healing is a lifelong process, one that is part of our task while living on Earth, our home for evolution, learning and service. Bailey described this healing presence (1970, p. 99):

> When man functions as a soul, he heals; he stimulates and vitalizes; he transmits the spiritual forces of the universe....Humanity's function is to transmit and handle force. This is done in the early and ignorant stages destructively and with harmful results. Later, when acting under the influence of the soul, force is rightly and wisely handled...more mercifully. Wholeness is its outcome.

As we support others with a spirit of compassion, the hallmark of nursing, we connect through our shared quality of love. Love is movement out of stillness, the movement of evolution. In this space we foster sharing, unfolding, flowering and becoming whole. Nursing gives us a vehicle to express these qualities, a way to share the energy of unconditional regard. Sharing is the ultimate movement of community, and only a world of sharing can be a peaceful and healthy world.

> *Patience is not waiting passively for something to happen,*
> *but is a kind of participation with the other in which we give*
> *fully of ourselves. It is misleading to understand patience*
> *simply in terms of time, for we give the other space as well.*
> *By patiently listening to the distraught person, by being present*
> *for them, we give them space to think and feel. Perhaps,*
> *instead of speaking of space and time, it would be truer to*
> *say that the patient person gives the other room to live;*
> *they enlarge the other's living room, whereas the impatient*
> *person narrows it.*
>
> Milton Mayeroff

Applying the Concepts in Nursing:

As a healing presence, you bear witness to the life and suffering of people you are privileged to care for. How well do you care for yourSelf? And how does your commitment to self-healing impact their own healing journey? The polarities that depict the level of development are listed below. They correspond to the seven chakra centers as well as the seven stages of healing. Evaluate these qualities of your own life:

SELF-CARE AND HEALING EXERCISE

Center 1: Safety and Security

Meeting your basic needs for survival and having what you need to feel confident in the world.

> *This perspective creates the necessary foundation for life and living. Activated at birth when the umbilical cord is cut, the vital energy system channels the life force into our body, creating a deep connection with the world. Associated with the root chakra at the base of tailbone (red), it energizes the physical body, lower extremities, including the feet, to establish and maintain your footing in the world. The mind-body begins by developing instrumental skills for survival, moving towards relational and imaginal skills fostering connection, curiosity, and creativity as we become more established in the world.*

Characteristics of this Stage

Starting Point	*Balanced*
Insecure and anxious	Confident and calm
Vulnerable and threatened	Secure and safe
Scarcity mentality	Abundance mentality
Isolated and self-conscious	Connected and self-reliant
Aggressive and manipulative	Disciplined and trustworthy

Checking In: To what extent (on a scale of 1–5):

- Do you feel safe?
- Do you feel trusting?
- Do you feel satisfied and fulfilled, irrespective of what you do?

- Do you sense abundance?
- Do you feel protected in the world?
- Do you financially secure?
- Do you feel accepted and part of the family/group/society?

Center 2: Strength and Vitality

Experiencing the joy of being vitally alive and fully engaged in a meaningful relationship with life through sensual and emotional fulfillment as well as creative expression.

> *This perspective activates all senses, providing sexual and creative energy as well as instinctual and emotional feelings. It boosts our awareness and desire for beauty, relationships and pleasure, establishing a healthy enthusiasm for being alive. Associated with the sacral chakra at the lower abdomen (orange), it energizes the reproductive organs, bladder and lower intestines. The intestines are a front line manager of infectious agents, and the general health of the immunosystem is fostered with the healthy maintenance of this center.*

Characteristics of this Stage

Starting Point	Balanced
Avoids or controls feelings	Embraces and honors feelings
Lives in head	Lives in whole body
Self-denies and self-neglects	Spontaneous and self-nurturing
Focus on work and productivity	Focus on life and self-expression
Lives in isolation	Lives in relationship

Checking In: To what extent (on a scale of 1–5):

- Do you pay attention to your body's signals and nurture them?
- Do you enjoy significant relationships?
- Do you pay attention to your feelings?
- Do you treat yourself gently?
- Do you celebrate the important occasions in life?
- Do you allow yourself little extravagances?
- Do you create beauty in life?

Center 3: Self-Esteem

Experiencing self-direction, physical energy, and personal expression of power and competency in life and career skills.

This perspective serves as a gateway for emotions and anger. Intellectually it influences our decision-making ability, sense of direction and personal power while emotionally it guides our ability to trust our most fundamental intuition and instincts. Our self-image and personality/ego are formed by the masks, characters and attitudes we adopt to navigate through the world, providing the determination, conviction and courage to achieve the life we are seeking. Associated with the solar plexus chakra at the naval (yellow), it energizes the spleen, adrenals, pancreas, stomach, upper intestines, gallbladder, liver, and lower back.

Characteristics of this Stage

Starting Point	*Balanced*
Defensive and Harsh	Patient and Gentle
Weak and Timid	Powerful and Strong
Directs and Suspects	Listens and Trusts
Workaholic overachiever	Balanced confidence
Victim mode	Partnership mode

Checking In: To what extent (on a scale of 1–5):

- Can you say no when appropriate?
- Are you able to make commitments and stick with them?
- Do you do as much for yourself as you do for others?
- Are you mutually respectful in your personal relationships?
- Are you able to stop disagreements before "blowing up" or getting excessively angry?
- Do you feel satisfied with the choices you are making in your life?
- Do you involve yourself with things that are important to you?

Center 4: Active Intelligence

Making choices with In-Sight! by integrating the body-mind with higher spiritual wisdom to gain In-Sight!

This perspective is the point of transformation, connecting the lower body-mind with higher soul wisdom. It serves as the center of balance for the entire physical/vital/mental system, fostering moral choices based on integrated information. Here we open our heart to connect with others in the spirit of altruism, compassion, generosity, empathy and caring. When balanced, we are able to open up, partake of and share with the Universe. Associated with the heart chakra at the center of chest (rose pink), it energizes the thymus, heart, circulatory system, breast, and blood flow.

Characteristics of this Stage

Starting Point	*Balanced*
Exclusive of others	Inclusive with others
Superior to others	Part of the human family
Righteous and judging	Compassionate and humble
Experiences ethnic divisions	Sees equality in diversity
Consistent struggle	Flow and Synchronicity

Of special note to "healers"—Other person's vital energy (non locally) often hits us at the heart chakra, especially when we are sympathetic. Empathy allows us to witness others suffering without taking it into our energy system.

Empathy Training for Professionals includes the following competencies:

1. Know yourself—learning to identify and feel your own emotions.

2. Practice emotional management—controlling your emotions in the motivation and service of your own goals.

3. Practice empathy—witnessing the emotions of others without identifying with them by maintaining your objectivity.

4. Manage emotional relationships—developing and maintaining good intrapersonal and interpersonal relationships over time.

Checking In: To what extent (on a scale of 1–5):

- Do you allow people to get close to you?
- Do you forgive easily?
- Do you naturally trust others?
- Are you light hearted?
- Do you enjoy helping others?
- Do you feel good about who you are?
- Are you naturally patient?

Center 5: Conscious Intention

Introducing our spirit to the world by living and articulating our life vision intentionally and authentically with compassion.

This center serves as the source for the motivation to fulfill our life purpose, as well as our ability for authentic self-expression. Our true intent, when aimed at serving the higher good, lays the foundation for trust, understanding, cooperation, and collaboration with others. Mindful self-expression is an agent for candid discussion, negotiation, and shared experiences in teaching and learning. Authentic presence fosters progress and evolution, peace, and healing relationships. Associated with our throat chakra at the back of neck (blue), it energizes the thyroid, parathyroid and hypothalamus, throat, neck, trachea, esophagus, mouth, teeth and ears.

Characteristics of this Stage

Starting Point	*Balanced*
Emphasizes appearance	Honesty in self expression
Difficulty conveying ideas	Expresses self with clarity
Focused on self-needs/desires	Focused on higher good for all
Controlling perfectionist	Accepting all perspectives
Over-intellectualizing	Balanced understanding

Checking In: To what extent (on a scale of 1–5):

- Are you mindful of what you say?
- Do you listen to others without interruption?
- Are you direct and forthright with grace?
- Are you truthful to yourself?
- Do people listen to you?
- Do you know what your expectations are?
- Do you care as much about the outcome for others as for yourself?

Center 6: Intuitive Innovation

Trusting our own inner wisdom acquired over many lifetimes while creating new ideas, and fresh solutions to existing challenges.

This perspective enhances quality of thought and all ways of knowing. It focuses our ability to see the abstract and subtle in life; to recognize hidden patterns, to perceive, understand, discern, dream, imagine, visualize and create. Imagination and the capacity for innovation create fertile soil for germination of new concepts, ideas and fantasies. The capacity for deep reflection helps us see the world and ourselves without distortion while opening our eyes to beauty and art as food for the soul. Associated with the brow chakra at the third eye between eyebrows (green), it energizes the pituitary gland, head, eyes, and all sense organs.

Characteristics of this Stage

Starting Point	Balanced
Muddled mind chatter	Intuitive knowing
Drone of confusion	Focused clarity
Influenced by logic	Influenced by insight
Taking things at face value	Seeing the deeper meaning
Guided by thinking and planning	Guided by inner knowing

Checking In: To what extent (on a scale of 1–5):

- Do you pay attention to subtle details and hidden aspects of a situation?
- Do you notice what others often overlook?
- Can you visualize something in your mind's eye in a flash of insight?
- Do you appreciate art and music, seeing them as essential in your life?
- Do you honor your intuition?
- Can you see into people and situations without judging appearances?
- Are you creative and inventive?

Center 7: Balanced Wholeness

Experiencing your highest wisdom and personal expression while bringing light to the world.

This perspective serves as the center for our highest spiritual consciousness and personal expression, connecting us to the source of Life. It opens the way for us to become a bearer of light in the world, focusing our attention on the spiritual meaning of life. Such a perspective begins to erase the imagined demarcation between what is and is not "me." A deep sense of community and desire to "give back" emerges, along with a grateful and generous countenance. Associated with the crown chakra at the top of head (gold), it energizes the pineal gland, brain stem, spinal cord, and nervous system.

Characteristics of this Stage

Starting Point	Balanced
Sees things in isolation	Sees all as interconnected
Restless and uncertain	Centered and peaceful
Confused about deep issues	Clear Self-knowing
Hyperactive and outspoken	Gentle and compassionate
Concerned about self	Community oriented

Checking In: To what extent (on a scale of 1–5):

- Do you have a sense that you are being watched over and cared for?
- Do you trust in the Divine order, synchronicity and miracles?
- Do you understand all life experiences as having a deep purpose?
- Do you believe that life is not a random event?
- Do you believe that all is well, no matter how it appears?
- Do you follow your inner guidance even when it doesn't make sense?
- Do you desire to "give back" to community?

A Living Example

Healing is a life-long journey. Sometimes when another is ill the healing is our own to do. When our daughter, Kristi, was so very ill, Wangi Waci made a "house call." After checking on Kristi, he came into the kitchen and asked me to articulate my greatest fear. I began to weep and confessed I feared that she was dying. He took one look at me, pointed to the door and said, "Get out of here and never come back. For whatever you think is possible for anyone is as far as they can go in your presence. Whether it is your children, spouse, patients, or colleagues, people become what you expect of them."

I thought of the countless ways in my life that I had judged others, sometimes harshly and other times out of pity. A parade of people in my recent and distant past began to march before my reflective sight. Then I began to recount the number of times I was misjudged, misrepresented, slighted by a careless gesture of another. Suddenly I got a deep knowing that we usually do not do this intentionally; it was the best or most conditioned response we knew it at that moment. Every time we get a new insight, a larger understanding, everything prior becomes only partial. New understandings do not reject but rather enlarge our understanding. It is important that we offer the same grace to ourselves as we begin to note and examine thoughts or behaviors that were less desirable.

Each thing, at its own time, is the best our capability can offer. When we start to show up to ourselves with this degree of honesty and nonjudgment, others can show up also. This is the beginning of compassion, for the world, and more difficultly, for ourselves. From that moment forward, I began to consciously work on my expectations of her, of myself, of every person and situation in my life. I invite you to do the same.

What do you expect from others and from yourself?

Web Site Resource: This website offers a framework that introduces, educates, and certifies the various aspects of holistic healing practices in nursing: *http://www.ahna.org/*

BIBLIOGRAPHY

Assagioli, R. (1992). *Psychosynthesis* (pp. 35–38). New York, NY: Anchor Books.

Bailey, A. A. (1970). *A treatise on white magic* (p. 99). New York, NY: Lucis Publishing.

Bendit, L. J. (1973). *The mysteries today* (p. 71). London, UK: The Theosophical Publishing House.

Bohm, D. (1980). *Wholeness and the implicate order* (p. 39). London, UK: Routledge & Kegan Paul.

Capra, F. (1988). *The tao of physics*. New York, NY: Bantam Books.

Chopra, D. (1993). *Ageless mind, timeless body*. New York, NY: Harmony Books.

Chopra, D. (2009). *Reinventing the body, resurrecting the soul*. New York, NY: Random House Publishing.

Dalai, Lama. (1986). *Health through balance*. Ithaca, NY: Snow Lion Publications.

Dossey, L. (1982). *Space, time and medicine*. Boulder, CO: Shambhala.

Dossey, L. (1993). *Healing words: The power of prayer and the practice of medicine*. New York, NY: HarperCollins Publisher.

Dossey, L. (2001). *Healing beyond the body* (p. 103). Boston, MA: Shambhala.

Dossey, L. (2008). Compassion and healing. In (Sounds True, ed.) *Measuring the Immeasurable: The scientific case for spirituality*. Boulder, CO: Sounds True.

Epstein, D. M. (1994). *The 12 stages of healing: A network approach to whole-ness*. San Rafel, CA: Amber-Allen Publishing.

Fisher, B. S. (1996). *Man, grand reflection of the greater cosmos: Studies in occult anatomy* (Vol. 3, pp. 75–78). Prescott, AZ: Subru Publications.

Goswami, A. (2004). *The quantum doctor: A physicist's guide to health and healing* (p. 226). Charlottesville, VA: Hampton Roads Publishing Company.

Koerner, J. (2004). *Mother heal myself: An intergenerational healing journey between two worlds*. Santa Rosa, CA: Crestport Press.

Kornfield, J. (1993). *A path with heart: A guide through the perils and promises of spiritual life*. New York, NY: Bantam Books.

Levine, P. (2008). Trauma and spirituality. In (Sounds True, ed.) *Measuring the immeasurable: The scientific case for spirituality* (pp. 85–100). Boulder, CO: Sounds True.

Lowen, A. (1980). *Depression and the body* (pp. 260–261, 267). New York, NY: Pelican Books.

Newman, M. (1986). *Health as expanding consciousness*. St. Louis, MO: C.V. Mosby Company.

Osho. (2003). *Mind-body balancing: Using your mind to heal your body*. New York, NY: St Martin's Griffin.

Pierrakos, J. (1987). *Core energetics* (p. 88). Mendocino, CA: LifeRhythm Publications.

Redfield, J. (1993). *The celestine prophecy*. Hoover, AL: Satori Publishing.

Roberts, B. (1985). *The path to no-self*. Boston, MA: Shambala, Publications.

Rogers, M. E. (1970). *An introduction to the theoretical basis of nursing*. Philadelphia, PA: F.A. Davis.

Schoch, M. (2005). *Healing with qualities*. Boulder, CO: Sentient Publications.

Siegel, D. (2008). Reflections on the Mindful Brain. In (Sounds True, ed.) *Measuring the immeasurable: The scientific case for spirituality*. Boulder, CO: Sounds True Publishing.

Talbot, M. (1986). *Beyond the quantum*. New York, NY: Macmillan.

Trungpa, C. (1984). *The sacred path of the warrior*. Boulder, CO: Shambhala Publications.

Walcott, D. (2001). *Uses of enchantment*. New York, NY: Vintage Books.

Yogananda, P. (1959). *Whispers for eternity*. Los Angles, CA: Self-Realization Fellowship.

Young, A. M. (1976). *The reflexive universe: Evolution of consciousness*. San Francisco, CA: Robert Briggs.

Zambucka, K. (1984). *The keepers of the earth*. Honolulu, HO: Harrame Publishing.

SECTION III

A HEALING PATH
WEAVING A PURPOSEFUL LIFE

*Life is a celebratory event.
Let us choose the forces of
life which will safeguard
the beauty of life.
Through hope, vision,
courage and will,
we create a purposeful life which
celebrates itself.*

Upanishads

CHAPTER 6

BALANCED LIVING
THE PATH OF BECOMING

Remember with gratitude the fruits of the labors of others,
Remember the beautiful things seen, heard and felt,
Remember the moments of distress that proved to be groundless,
Remember the new people met who teach true character and
*   human dignity,*
Remember the dreams who keep us ever mindful of hopes
*   and goals which inspire,*
Remember the Spirit of the One who seeks us out in our
*   aloneness,*
Who gives a sense of assurance that undercuts despair
And confirms life with new courage and abiding hope.

Howard Therman

Our being, the very essence of our life, is in a constant state of change. We are tangible. Unique. Present. Embodied. Evolving! And we are witnessing a great mystery; the discovery of the self-organizing, self-synthesizing, and infinitely creative process moving through the cosmos—and ourselves. As we truly grasp the power of the ever unfolding and evolving Spirit of the Universe, we realize that we are on sacred ground. Although we recognize that we are in charge of our individual destiny, we often forget that we are also part of a larger, eternal human and universal destiny. In reality, we are not separate from each other, from nature, or Spirit. Universal Spirit connects the inner and outer being of all in a continuous and ever-changing dance of life.

Nursing is a profession called into being by the society it serves. We come to our work with a noble purpose, the aspiration for service. Supporting others facing a health challenge or a

175

life passage such as birth and death requires us to take ourselves out of the center and put spirit in our place. Although we cannot fully understand or describe spirit, Fetzer Institute has crafted a description intended not to be definitive but rather to be framing for shared consideration (Lehman, 2004, pp. 11–13):

> By spirit we mean the Universal Spirit that is the deepest and most inclusive ground of being. Spirit is the source of all that exits. Spirit is the infinite, creative energy that gives birth to the universe. Spirit is the common source of the world's faith traditions. Spirit is the love that creates and sustains life.

It is the spiritual values of compassion and caring that unite our nursing mission and identity. Healing and wholeness emerge from the spirit orientation of our service. Together we draw upon the scientific, educational, and religious/philosophical resources that free the powers of love, forgiveness, and healing that reside in every human being.

The field and object perspective of wholeness observes life as a complimentary dance of being and doing, outer and inner, a path of choicelessness, and also of choice. We like to choose because we enjoy being in control. Paradoxically, we make choices within the context of a choiceless existence. We did not choose our parents, our culture, or language, at lease consciously. However, we did choose our profession, our significant relationships, and the manner in which we approach life. Total emphasis on choice leads to anxiety, while adherence to choicelessness leads to passivity. It is the appropriate mix and movement between our acceptance of choicelessness and the dynamism of choice that creates the most vibrant dance of life.

Choiceless things must be accepted unconditionally to bring harmony to our lives. We are human beings, calling us to an unconditional acceptance of the human family. We are also made of spirit and unconditional love, so it is not an optional extra. Love is choiceless, but the ways we choose to express it are optional. Choicelessness is not fatalism; it is not passive. It is an active acceptance of reality—an "isness." It is getting into alignment with our being, our vocation, our destiny. From that context, we make choices through the expression of our creativity, imagination, and improvisational capacity (Kumar, 2004, pp. 32–35).

The unity of life manifests in millions of forms, but each form makes our own particular contribution to the movement of the whole. We are born with our own unique gifts, the essence of our natural self. The complimentarity of "being" and "doing" flows out of our authentic self. Therefore, choices that are not made out of our true identity will inevitably lead us astray.

Nurses who walk in dynamic balance are in touch with their authenticity. A balanced life is a life of authentic alignment. They receive whatever is given to them from the process of the universe and the natural order as a gift. Received with gratitude and joy rather than struggle and resistance, they flow in harmony with the natural order. From that context, conscious choices are made regarding the particulars that enhance their life journey in a manner that fulfills the destiny of their soul.

EXPANDING CONSCIOUSNESS—A SHIFT TOWARD AUTHENTICITY

We journey in two worlds simultaneously. The outer world is visible, tangible, and observed by the masses. Nothing is hidden, except from ourselves when we choose to marginalize or ignore things painful or difficult. The inner world, however, is a mysterious place filled with fears, fantasies, and thoughts bigger than life. We are both drawn to and afraid of what lies at the depth of our being. Often we believe that this world is invisible to the naked eye, known only to us in quiet moments alone. However, nothing could be further from the truth. Just as our personality demonstrates our style of moving through the world, our values portray our inner world of thoughts, beliefs, and expectations that focus our efforts and energy, betraying illusions of secrecy and anonymity. By watching and listening to a person, all is revealed.

Values: Guide to Personal and Professional Development

Values are a reflection of consciousness: they reveal the activity and attention of the Focus Point of our mind. Values are symbols, a shorthand word that identifies what inspires us, what empowers us, and what prompts us to act. Values are the driving force and motivation for the choices and actions that guide our life.

Although chaos and emergence of new order are nonlinear phenomenon, predictable patterns and fractals are also part of the quantum world. Looking closely at our evolutionary path, behavioral theorists have identified specific patterns of development

Basic Tenets on Values

I-Values reflect your beliefs, attitudes, and expectations, directing the priorities you live by.

- They focus your attention, influencing what you see.
- They filter thoughts that influence how you interpret things and the meaning ascribed.
- They guide the choices and actions that direct your life.

II-Values guide consciousness development.

- Consciousness is an ever-evolving phenomenon at the cellular/individual/cosmic level.
- Continuous development occurs at physical/social/spiritual levels of being.
- Values cluster into certain areas of focus to help us accomplish a developmental task.
- Within each developmental task are various skill sets that prepare you for the next cycle of growth:
  - Technical life skills
  - Relationship abilities
  - Reasoning capacities
- Lived experience expands your awareness, moving the focus to a higher level of values-guided development.
- Each stage enlarges your circle of relationships along with a greater sense of autonomy, accountability, and authenticity.
- Every stage actualizes your potential more fully.

III-Values are a reflection of your conscious awareness, your level of energetic vibration.

- They reflect your understanding of how the world works.
- Each values-focused level expands your understanding of the universe and your relationship with it.
- Increased awareness broadens your capacity to respond and co-create rather than reacting from a base of conditioned expectations.
- Ethical behavior is of necessity conscious behavior.

IV-Values bifurcate into two domains.

Personal/Individual Values- (BEING—your Inner World of beliefs and aspirations)

- Developed/Influenced by choices and thoughts
- Satisfy the need for creation of meaning

(continued)

Basic Tenets on Values (continued)

- Every individual has a set of core values that establishes personal parameters—often unexamined and unconscious—rules for living.
- While family play a large role in defining personal values in infancy and childhood, development across the lifespan enlarges and deepens core values/authenticity.
- Living our values with intention maintains our priorities and life focus.

Workplace/Shared Values (DOING—your Outer World of opportunities and experiences)

- Developed/influenced by relationships and contribution.
- Satisfy the need for life experience.
- Every organization/community has a set of core values that establish cultural parameters—often unspoken and unwritten—rules for working together.
- While leaders play a large role in defining organizational culture by their actions and leadership, all employees contribute to the culture within their own unit or department.
- A shared values-based culture holds the key to employee loyalty and commitment.
- Shared professional values are the unifying energy for the discipline.

V-Shared Values respond to their surroundings.

- While individual values are consistent, shared values are influenced by the culture/environment
- The Focal Point shifts in response to the situation or relationship in which you find yourself
  - Your energy influences those around you
  - When higher energy prevails, individuals may move into a values stage beyond their current capacity
  - When lower energy prevails, individuals may succumb to negative pressure
- Hierarchy of needs will direct the Focal Point to the appropriate stage/level
  - Maintaining a predominant Outer World focus, or stalling, may occur if one is faced with a difficult life challenge
  - When security is threatened, individuals revert to values of safety
- Congruence between personal and professional values increases career satisfaction and effectiveness, decreasing burnout, turnover and poor performance.

from infancy through adulthood Barrett (1998), Benner (1984), Erikson (1980), Drucker (1999), Maslow (1980), Hall (1986), and Rogers (1980). The model builds upward from a solid base:

Seven Stages of Values-Guided Development

Tier Seven: SELF-ACTUALIZATION—Love and Unity
(Universal Identity—Self-Knowledge)
Integration Skills
Examples: Forgiveness Humility Compassion Beauty Spirituality

Tier Six: WISDOM—Intuition and Creativity
(Creative Identity—Self-Expression)
Imaginal Skills
Examples: Innovation Insight Wisdom Adaptability Emotional
Intelligence

Tier Five: INTENTION—Purpose and Goals
(Archetypal Identity—Self-Reference)
Reflective Skills
Examples: Authenticity Service Caring Make a Difference Community
Involvement

Tier Four: ACTIVE INTELLIGENCE—Analytic and Abstract
(Self-Expression—Social Identity)
Implementation Skills
Examples: Flexibility Collaboration Patience Humor/Fun Problem
Solving

Tier Three: SELF ESTEEM—Skill and Power
(Self-Definition—Ego Identity)
Vocational Skills
Examples: Trust Competence Efficiency Autonomy Professional
Growth

Tier Two: RELATIONSHIPS—Belonging and Vitality
(Self-Discovery—Emotional Identity)
Interpersonal Skills
Examples: Passion Honesty Respect Laughter/Play Family

Tier One: SAFETY—Physical and Psychological
(Self-Preservation—Physical Identity)
Instrumental Skills
Examples: Responsible Health Dependable Fairness Order

FIGURE 6.1

Values-Guided Development Model

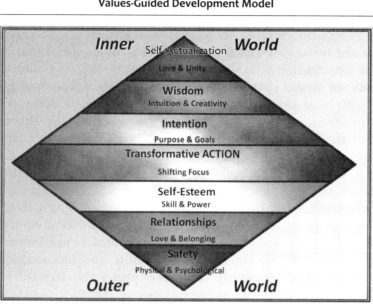

In nested fashion, each stage has specific tasks to be accomplished that prepare us for the next phase (Figure 6.1). Messy and wandering, our path is not a linear, one-size-fits-all journey. Forces, inner and outer, are always at play, making the journey an adventure of magnitude.

VALUES STAGE MODEL

Once we have more or less completed a seven-stage cycle, it repeats at higher levels of complexity, refining our capacity as we now have a full range of basic values to draw from in each situation encountered. Values-guided development increasingly progresses from an Outer World to an Inner World focus.

Our journey is a continuous dance between "doing" and "being," the evolution of spirit ever moving forward. The first three stages of values focus on our capacity to relate to the Outer World with a focus on "doing." The final three stages focus on development of the Inner World with a deepening capacity for "being." A solid foundation in the Outer World establishes a framework for developing a strong Inner World whose values foster a creative and compassionate presence. Dynamic balance occurs when these two worlds meet in the middle ground to guide authentic and life-giving choices. The ability to shift focus between the two worlds increasingly brings all of ourSelf to any situation. We increase ability to surf between Inner and Outer by expanding our capacity for Active Intelligence.

Outer World is the first to be developed. A concrete physical body must establish a safe foundation from which to move through the world. Therefore, choices and actions are externally referenced in the first three stages. Children rely on the rules of family, authority figures, and the culture that supports life and livelihood, responding and/or reacting to what they are told. Young professionals will look to expert clinicians who have a successful and proven past as they navigate the entry into their career. We are all testing a foundation built by others, evaluating what does and does not work for "me," what is and what is not "my truth." This creates the foundation for our reliable and predictable self, which is the dependable and competent personality/ego the world comes to know and expect (Coles, Erikson, 2000).

Inner World begins to reveal itself as our growing awareness strengthens our sense of "self" and our own knowledge gleaned from ever broadening lived experience. Choices become increasingly internally referenced. When we begin to recognize and connect with our authentic self, we become clear about our true intent. At this point, energetically our vibration is of sufficient frequency to open our intuition—the doorway to our soul.

Our soul holds the blueprint for our unique destiny. It also contains all of the abilities, relationship, and experiences required to actualize our authentic presence, our unique contribution to the world. We begin to use our Spiritual Ego, which coordinates inner wisdom and creativity with an intention for higher good in responding to life events. Synchronicity, experienced as flow, brings us the right situations and relationships to help create a reality we desire as our increased vibrational frequency attracts what is appropriate. The Focal Point of "middle ground" increasingly shifts between the two worlds but begins with the voice of intuitive inner wisdom rather than external ego. Logic is added to perception, not the other way around. Our decisions become more inclusive, more impactful, and more life giving for all. Life becomes a joyful journey, irrespective of outer circumstances in the world (Choquette, 2000).

Deeper Wisdom—The Gift of In-Sight!

Moving beyond fixation on physical existence in the external world into an equally daring and disciplined exploration of our inner life crosses a threshold into the landscape of the soul and transcendence, leading to personal and global transformation. Our unfolding story is influenced by the genes that make up the human body and by natural instincts that trigger an action below the level of conscious awareness. Our choices and decisions, however, are strongly influenced by the values acquired in our cultural heritage. This system codes "appropriate" behavior, often limiting us to conduct better suited for some past time. Recognition of the forces and choices that limit our journey toward increasing consciousness and human capacity makes it possible to become liberated from them (Thuman, 2004).

As children, we encounter developmental experiences, which make us acutely aware of how to navigate the outer world. Rules of family, experiences, and activities inform and reinforce our understanding of the world and our place in it. In logical fashion, we create mental models of right and wrong from a learned set of values that are intended to protect, manage, direct, and acquire what we want or need in the world of *"me"* in the *Outer World of "Form."*

The turbulent onset of adolescence fosters increasing response to another information source, our inner wisdom. Intent coupled with imagination starts to push past the rules of society, responding with greater sensitivity to the intuitive promptings of the soul. In silent reflection, purpose and meaning are generated, tested, evaluated, and integrated into our expanding world view. This activity arises from a set of values that are collective in nature, directed toward what is needed for *"we"* in the *Inner World of "Awareness."*

The unifying field for these worlds is the *World of Mind*: our true home. More powerful than genetic origin or geographic residence, the dwelling place of mind connects our inner and outer worlds. The dilemma of a purely reasoning mind is that it hinders the perception of the complex beauty of true reality. As events occur our intuition spontaneously sees them as they are, while the mind interprets and forms mental constructs about them. Perception by intuition coming from the soul is direct and instantaneous, and it knows by direct and clear observation. The mind, however, goes through an elaborate process couched within the limitations of its scope of awareness. It takes what it sees and filters it through lifelong conditioning and acquired perspectives, that is, the politician's perceptions are colored by political agendas, predetermined policies, and party loyalty.

Over time, orderly patterns of observation are collected in our subconscious mind. The more the patterns fit together, the more we come to know about the phenomenon they represent. The closer we zoom in on a single fact, the more the pattern of the whole is blurred. Every "fact" is only one part of a larger pattern— what we really understand is the pattern. To fully grasp any situation, we need sensory data analyzed by reason and logic, plus we need to intuit how the pattern holds together. From this flash of recognition, we grasp the pattern as a whole.

In-Sight! occurs in the freedom of being liberated from deeply held beliefs, well-worn grooves of thought about how the world works, who and what we are, and what it means to be in relationship with each other and the larger world. To find deeper meaning in our lives and more comprehensive solutions to current dilemmas, we need to combine our thoughts with inner wisdom. A balanced approach to life occurs when we honor both aspects of knowing.

Active Intelligence incorporates wisdom and creative capacity as focus shifts between our inner and outer world throughout the day. Awareness and activity begin with the authentic self rather than an ego-guided role identity. Here one identifies intent; "why am I doing this and what do I hope to accomplish or contribute?" One also draws deeply from imagination and creativity; "while I know this is the current practice, how else might this be accomplished or improved?"

A logical and reliable person uses past experience and personal expectations to guide and direct the competing demands of the day:

In this "normal" state of awareness, we identify with our thought processes, reactions, desires, and aversions. Run by the ego, we are in a continuous low level of unease, discontent, boredom, or nervousness—a constant background static of inner pollution. The more we are ruled by standards, norms, and requirements, the less we hear those soft intuitive whispers from deep within our authentic and creative soul.

Cycle of Logic—The Outer World

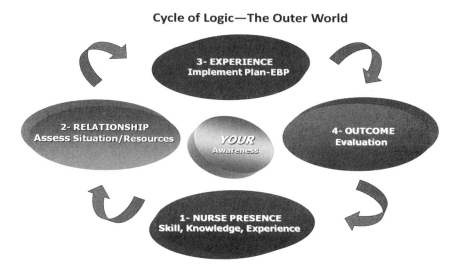

Instead of performing from a learned script, an "authentic person" begins with an intuitive, unprogrammed approach to life:

Cycle of Intuition—The Inner World

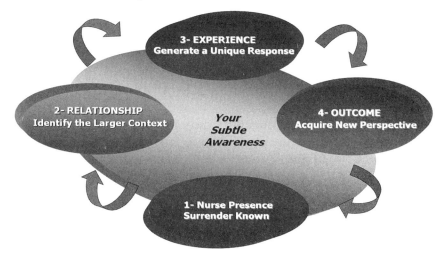

The larger situation becomes visible when we truly step into the moment-NOW. As we learn to witness our own thoughts, expectations and emotions, rather than being driven by them, we become surprised at their influence.

Anything unconscious becomes conscious as we turn our focus toward it; the truth of the moment stands out clearly. Instead of looking for the standard-based evidence, we see what is present. Instead of listening for the expected, we hear what is meant behind the words. Once clear about the uniqueness of the situation and the people involved, we then draw on the strong foundation of our past experience, expectation, and expertise to deal with the issue at hand. We are fortified, not limited by our past, and all is elevated to a higher order; synchronicity becomes the norm.

Choices that begin from deep within guide us to become more authentic and transparent in our self-expression. We start bringing creativity, flexibility, and playfulness to the moment. We increasingly test the requests and perspectives of others; taking broader risks while collaborating in an innovative fashion. We begin to share our viewpoints with others, co creating part of the "evidence-based practice" that others refer to as they begin their own transformative journey.

Tapping into the deeper levels of being where our true innate intelligence resides requires bringing the spiritual dimension into the healing process. As we integrate our inner world and rhythms into our life, we begin to experience a flowing interconnectedness around us, which eventually includes the entire human and planetary family.

PRACTICING WITH MASTERY—
PERSONAL AND PROFESSIONAL BALANCE

Professional mastery encompasses more than clinical competence: it includes a moral, ethical, and caring presence that performs the role of nurse in a comprehensive and inclusive manner (Leonard, 1992). Mastery is not perfection but rather a journey, and the true master must be willing to try and fail and try again. To a large extent, the kind of professional a person becomes depends on the strength of their personal foundation. The professional self emerges from the personal through values, intent, beliefs, and goals that inform and guide their clinical choices and actions.

The complexities of the 21st-century health care system demand dynamic and vibrant nurses who provide service and compassion to the public. The one essential quality of today's professional is that they must be their own person, authentic in every regard.

Nurses are professional knowledge workers whose wisdom falls into several domains:

- *Nursing Science*: Knowledge for clinical care and safety
  - Ability to understand scientific laws and principles
  - Ability to analyze and evaluate
  - Ability to bring logic and reason to decision making
  - Ability to make judgments and conclusions from relevant data
- *Nursing Art*: Knowledge for understanding
  - Ability to analyze the current situation from multiple perspectives
  - Ability to recognize and comprehend the subtle patterns underlying the phenomenon being viewed
  - Ability to join and integrate seemingly unrelated parts into a larger whole
  - Ability to synthesize findings into creation of new order
- *Nursing Presence*: Knowledge for witnessing and creation of meaning
  - Ability to identify subtle energetic connections
  - Ability to grasp significance and meaning unfolding for the client
  - Ability to witness without interference in client's process
  - Ability to conduct oneself in a moral manner

A knowledge professional whose style is consistent with their personality and character is autonomous, highly independent, practices with solid values, develops enduring relationships, and leads from the heart. Such a nurse demonstrates self-discipline, identifies their own growth edge, and continues to develop skills and capacities while integrating them into a unified whole.

Values development continues across the life span and, for nurses, can be categorized into two dimensions: personal and professional. The predominant value clusters between the two worlds create a specific pattern of self-management, which fosters an explicit leadership style in their personal and organizational life:

- *Personal Values*: Those values that guide and shape our inner landscape of beliefs and aspirations. They guide our thoughts and choices, satisfying our basic needs for connection and meaning

FIGURE 6.2

Nurse Values Profile Exemplar

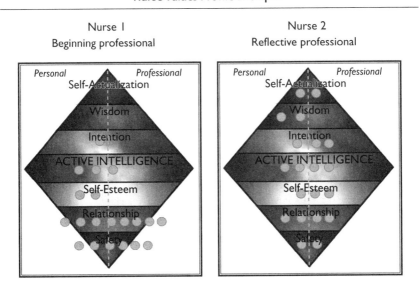

Nurse 1
Beginning professional

Nurse 2
Reflective professional

- *Professional Values*: Those values that guide and shape our external world of work and society. They guide our relationships and workplace actions, satisfying our basic needs for contribution and community
- *Leadership Style*: The unique clustering of values in both the personal and professional domains giving rise to a certain pattern of self-management and leadership that are manifest in our private and organizational life

A healthy individual moves easily from one environment to the other, as life circumstances demand. However, if we have not developed the core capacities in a specific values stage, we are destined to go back to complete that developmental task or continue to experience challenges when we get "stuck" in that specific area (Izzo & Withers, 1996).

The development of the professional self follows the same sequence that the personal self experiences. Specific tasks achieved in sequential order lead to the evolving sense of authenticity, mastery, and wholeness. Research suggests that it takes approximately

3 years to develop mastery of basic nursing practice, and then the nurse becomes a guide for others (Benner, 1984; Benner, Tanner, & Chesla, 1996).

The following seven stages of professional development have been identified as essential for a healthy and vibrant professional practice (Leddy & Pepper, 1989; Erikson, 1980; Mezirow & Associates, 1991):

- *Launching Professional*—Focuses on skills
- *Beginning Professional*—Focuses on fit
- *Young Professional*—Focuses on identity
- *Growing Professional*—Focuses on independence
- *Reflective Professional*—Focuses on collaboration
- *Maturing Professional*—Focuses on contribution
- *Older Professional*—Focuses on completion

The quality of goal achievement in one stage will strongly influence movement to the next level. Successful completion of each stage greatly influences later role achievement. Although it is important to focus on clinical skill competency (especially in the first three stages of professional development), equally important are other aspects of role development. It is process-oriented skills such as communicating, evaluating, educating, collaborating, and advocating that guide and enlarge clinical understanding and engagement with the patient and others on the health team. The addition of energy-focused skills of active observation and active receptivity, combined with active intelligence, creates a more comprehensive skill set for the postmodern nurse. Expanding competency in inquiry and experimentation, comfort with ambiguity, clarity in communication, and decisive and moral action, is the hallmark of a reflective practitioner (Mezirow & Associates, 1991).

Personal–Professional Development Exemplar

Using the values profiling tool developed in conjunction with the American Association of Critical Care Nurses and the American Home Health Association (refer to chapter 10), the following values profiles and weighted values cluster were obtained (Bodensteiner, 2001).

The values profile of the two following nurses is reflective of their level of professional development and their experiences in the world:

● Nurse 1 is a 21-year-old female with an ADN in Nursing, who is in the sixth month of her first career experience. Her values profile shows major focus on activities surrounding building a solid foundation in both personal and professional aspects of her life. Her values clustered at a Stage 3 level of development.
● Nurse 2 is a 54-year-old female with a Diploma in Nursing, who is in the 32nd year of her career. Her values profile shows a well-balanced profile in both the personal and professional domains, with a values clustering at Stage 5.

Analysis of each profile tells much about the essence of each nurse as we examine:

● *Values Stages*: A clustering of related values reflects a stage of development with defining characteristics regarding overall level of conscious awareness. The next stage can be attained by establishing and pursuing growth strategies for further maturation and development, if our life experiences are embraced and reviewed for the learning that they offer.
  ● *Values Gap*: Occasionally, a level of personal or professional development has no identified values. When the gap is in only one dimension of our life, it may be something unconsciously taken care of or it is moving toward the next stage of growth. If the gap is consistent in both the personal and professional domain, it may indicate an unfinished developmental task that may show up under stress and could be revisited and completed.
  ● *Values Congruence*: Personal values are dictated by the soul, while professional values flow from within the discipline. They are also influenced by the patient population served, the culture of the working environment, and values of the leadership within the organization. Having some values that bridge both worlds leads to greater congruence in our life and greater satisfaction in our work.

The values that comprise these seven centers are initially developed during the first phase of life, with modification and refinement occurring as we continue to revisit these issues repeatedly across the lifespan (Lewis, 1991).

Each profile is an exquisite picture of a life in progress. It is a graphic depiction of the various stages of development we master during a meaningful career. It also demonstrates the dynamic possibilities for a continuing evolution toward mastery when we engage deeply with life.

HEALING THE PROFESSION—FROM WITHIN

While our story is filled with incredible acts of caring and compassion, we also hold the collective memory of systematic oppression and gender discrimination. Nursing has a long and challenging history around its relationships with physicians, health care organizations, and one another (Achterberg, 1990).

Human evolution is replete with a history of widespread trauma and wounding. Our "collective consciousness" carries the burden of hundreds of millions of people who have experienced the ravages of genocide, human rights violations, and racial and ethnic conflicts. Simultaneously, in the past 5 years, new wars, violence, neglect, and weather disasters have added millions of others to the toll of those scarred and wounded (Thompson & O'Dea, 2005).

New ideas and initiatives focused on addressing the intractable conflicts and complex social intergenerational wounds are emerging in every sector of society. There is a global awakening for the need to transition from violence and massive social wounding toward building a framework for a culture committed to peace and wholeness.

Nursing is situated in a strategic position to assist with the social healing of a fractured world in general and our own discipline in particular. Following the tragedy of 9/11, many parents called in to TV children's show host Mr. Rogers, asking how to help their child. His immediate response was, "keep them focused on the helpers."

Healing of an individual, a discipline, or a world begins with the recognition of the role that mind "consciousness" plays in the recovery process. Just as medical research has demonstrated the link between mind (thoughts, feelings, and emotions) and body, social healing views the communal "group mind" as critical to moving forward. Energetically we share commonly held images, attitudes, beliefs, and collective traumas, which are instrumental in shaping and creating either the repetitive feedback loop of victim/perpetrator or liberation from it. The work of social healing helps to soften the well-worn identity frames that keep us bound in outworn spaces.

Social (nursing-feminine) wounds are held in the "social body"—a shared structure of meaning that bonds the group together energetically. As a result, if true healing is to occur, there must be a transformation of consciousness, a new way of understanding at the personal level, the context, content, and possibilities for reconciliation concerning the phenomenon. Simultaneously, this must be accompanied by a system-wide transformation of the organizations in which we are nested. The process must be both interactive and interdependent. This calls for an intrinsically holistic approach to social healing, by addressing both its structural and spiritual dimensions (Rifkin, 2009).

The health of our discipline, the health of society, and the earth who sustains us all must take into account all dimensions of our global traumas, from the personal to the political, from the biological to the spiritual. True social healing will require change on many levels. We must explore structures of economics, politics, regulation, and justice, along with social and cultural aspects of the health care field. Simultaneously, we must stay alert to the quality of our individual awareness, our own expressions of compassion in action, the truth of our interdependence, and how we contribute to it (Thurman, 2004).

Social position (race/education/economic status), privilege, and power are "concerns of the spirit" that must be considered. While we explore central issues with people of power, we must be equally aware of our own attitudes toward and relationship with the many multiskilled workers who carry out support services that assist our daily practice. How do we honor, respect, and interact with those who are "not us?"

When our daughter was deep into the struggle of her near-death experience, in the healing ceremony the Medicine Man

*identified our five-generation history of death in childbirth.
It was later mentioned that he 'saw' the energetic pictures
in my auric field. He then went on to explain that patriarchal
oppression from cultural/religious beliefs were a root cause. If
I wanted my daughter to heal I would simply have to 'forgive'
all male oppression in the world. I staggered backward and
fell against the tree as the weight of his request crushed me to
the very fiber of my being. "How could I begin such a daunting task?" I whispered as visions of difficult experiences with
physicians, administrators, authority figures in my personal life
began to flow in unceasing succession. He chuckled and said,
"Oh, that's easy! Just forgive yourself for all the times that you
have oppressed others." I thought of the many ways, large and
small, that I had truly done that very thing to others, and felt
the searing shame of recognition of my own contribution to
the cause of world oppression. From that flash of insight—
everything changed. And in that new knowing, I healed an old
wound, releasing judgment and resentment on many levels. It
helped me focus my attention to forgiveness, of others—and
more importantly and difficulty—myself. It was an initiation
into compassion, and becoming a healing presence at the bedside of my beloved daughter. We are one with all that
surrounds us.*

Nursing is a universal phenomenon. The global field of nursing
can stand together as we extend the responsibility for healing our
collective professional wound to the greater whole. However, we
must be mindful of the impact that our own privileges may have
on others. We must understand the implications of coming from
a society with a context for power that includes a legacy of sys-
temic imbalances created through a history of slavery, genocide of
native peoples, discriminatory policies, and an ongoing mentality
of punitive and retributive actions including war and incarcera-
tion. Truth and reconciliation are crucial to understand in every
context of our lives.

New understandings occur through a shared dialogue of
the heart. Such encounters reveal that space in between, where a
greater knowing and truth reside. Upon the ending of Apartheid in
Africa, Desmond Tutu observed that retribution closes any chance
for a future. Reconciliation, on the other hand, opens the door for
tomorrow. Transitioning from the age-old issues of oppression that
have plagued our profession for so long is no easy journey. This

complex healing journey requires finding the balance between truth and justice, peace and mercy. It is a multigenerational task rather than an immediate fix. In the end, *it is a task for each one of us to accomplish personally.* We are then in a position to offer new insights, create a deeper conversation, and give birth to new models and metaphors that will restore wholeness to the profession and the field. Only then will nursing as a collective service offer a truly healing presence to the world.

> When we learn to trust the deep resources of our own being, we discover more than simple renewal. We begin to touch the place where the universe is alive with fresh insight, new possibilities, and supportive resources for realizing our highest ideals. This inner resource flows from an alignment of both heart and mind, making a commitment to the collective human journey through a science of being that flows from an open heart and mind. This generates a positive path for human evolution and genuine progress on planet Earth.
>
> *Unknown Teacher*

Applying the Concepts in Nursing

The development of the professional self follows the same sequence that the personal self experiences. Specific developmental tasks to be achieved at each stage of professional development are listed, along with a Check In Quiz to test your perception regarding what comprises the "developmental task" and how well you have accomplished it for yourself. Development of clinical competence, process and presence skills fosters an evolving sense of authenticity, mastery, and wholeness.

PROFESSIONAL DEVELOPMENT ANALYSIS

Stage 1—Launching Professional—Focus on Skill

The goals of a new nurse entering practice are to develop trust in one's preceptors and managers, to effectively develop their abilities to fulfill professional role requirements, to be able to count on others to assist them in meeting patient objectives, to experience gratification in their new role, and to receive recognition for a job well done.

Characteristics of this Stage:

Productive:

- Trusts in self and team members with strong sense of accomplishment
- Focuses energy on meeting client needs with confidence
- Optimistic regarding professional opportunities across career

Nonproductive:

- Mistrusts self and professional peers with guarded relationships
- Doubts own competency with energy focused on meeting own needs
- Focuses on short-term tasks versus long-range goals

Checking In: To what extent (on a scale of 1–5)

- Do you feel educationally prepared for this work?
- Do you feel self-sufficient and competent?
- Do you find risk-taking increasingly easier?
- Do you feel clear and confident when asked to make a client care decision?
- Do you get others to get things done without the need to manipulate or coerce them?
- Do you understand and meet the needs and expectations of the client and family?
- Do you feel supported in your work environment?

Stage 2—Beginning Professional—Focus on Fit

After successful initiation into the profession, the goals expand: to depend on more mature professionals for guidance some of the time, to experience self as a professional in their own right, to know that others on the team value their presence and their contribution, to admit that "not knowing so let's find out" is a sign of strength rather than weakness.

Characteristics of this Stage:

Productive:

- Trusts self as competent and knowledgeable
- Trusts client's wisdom regarding their own care
- Develops effective interpersonal relationships that demonstrate collaboration

Nonproductive:

- Views self as servant who "carries out" orders give by others
- Views client as subordinate versus partner in care team
- Maintains procedural focus

Checking In: To what extent (on a scale of 1–5)

- Do you have the necessary education and information to understand and meet the changing needs of the client?
- Are you skilled in establishing, maintaining, and terminating a therapeutic relationship?
- Do you understand the rules and culture of the unit and organization?
- Do you communicate clearly, effectively, and appropriately with colleagues and supervisors?
- Do you respect and express your intelligence and feelings appropriately with clients and families?
- Do you work well within a team, knowing when to lead, delegate, or when to follow?
- Do you feel comfortable and competent around the patient?

Stage 3—Young Professional—Focus on Identity

The young professional now experiences a deeper sense of competency in the role, seeks experiences to independently expand their knowledge in a specific area of practice, and seeks a mentor to learn the wisdom of a master rather than textbook learning. A nurse at this stage is ideal as a preceptor to RNs new to the field or those returning after an extended period away from the practice. Participation in unit-based projects facilitates organizational skill development at this stage.

Characteristics of this Stage:

Productive:

- Offers creative ideas for development of alternatives in problem solving
- Takes risks in carrying out advocacy role for client—accepting accountability for decisions and actions
- Begins to share newfound wisdom through preceptor role with new graduates and young professionals

Nonproductive:

- Relies on policy rather than taking initiative
- Seeks reward for efficiency versus sound judgment and is more comfortable with routine than independent decisions
- Accountable to employer rather than client

Checking In: To what extent (on a scale of 1–5)

- Do you help the client identify their long-term concerns and create strategies to reach desired outcomes?
- Are you able to communicate your needs clearly and honestly?
- Do you allow others to be unhappy or uncomfortable without trying to rescue them?
- Do you have a realistic view of patient rights and organizational capacity?
- Do you address authority figures with your observations openly and freely?
- Do you identify and meet the learning needs of the client?
- Do you participate in nursing research studies and apply findings to your practice?

Stage 4—Growing Professional—Focus on Independence

Professional identity is enlarging along with a personal belief system about the discipline of nursing; skill in area of specialty practice expands, and competency in experimentation is leading to an expanding awareness of the nursing role in implementing planned change through partnerships and teamwork. A nurse at this stage of development serves in an expanding clinical practice role, as a charge nurse or as a preceptor to experienced nurses returning to school.

Characteristics of this Stage:

Productive:

- Expands professional network to increase competency
- Demonstrates behavior promoting initiative rather than conformity
- Seeks continuing education to further develop role rather than out a sense of duty

Nonproductive:

- Feels inadequate rather than professionally competent
- Feels "other directed" rather than "self-directed"
- Feels others control practice, so has "no time" for professional tasks as assigned procedural tasks consume all the time available

Checking In: To what extent (on a scale of 1–5)

- Do you turn an unpleasant situation into a pleasant one?
- Do you take offense?
- Do you coordinate the efforts of multiple health care workers providing care?
- Do you promote the client's ability to act more independently?
- Do you admit weaknesses and mistakes readily and access resources to remediate them?
- Do you speak out when you are asked to do something you don't believe in?
- Are you generous in giving support and encouragement?

Stage 5—Reflective Professional—Focus on Collaboration

Professional identity now expands from independence to interdependence with clients, peers, and other colleagues in the health care delivery system; mutual assessment of total needs of client, family, and community; awareness and respect for the unique contributions of each discipline, determining who is best qualified for the aspect of care required; evaluation of the health care system including policy and reward structures. Beginning leadership positions as well as mentor role with other experienced professionals occurs at this level of development.

Characteristics of this Stage:

Productive:

- Values clinical practice and serves as a mentor to other nurses
- Initiates discovery and learning, continuously engaged as a consumer of research findings, and contributes to the literature
- Positively impacts society's image of nursing through role modeling behavior

Nonproductive:

- Leaves client with experience of nursing as attendant and mechanical rather than professional and dynamic
- Creates a public image of nursing as technical with restorative care as only the focus
- Leaves profession feeling burned out and unfulfilled, having missed multiple opportunities within the profession

Checking In: To what extent (on a scale of 1–5)

- Are you creative and adaptable?
- Do you identify common meanings in a group conflict that identify the core issue?
- Do you care as much about other people's development as your own?
- Are you direct and forthright in receiving and giving feedback, with grace?
- Are you a good communicator and negotiator?
- Do people have confidence in you?
- Do you organize and manage a task by dividing and delegating its various components?

Stage 6—Maturing Professional—Focus on Contribution

The maturing professional develops goals for others in nursing, contributing to society through efforts in nursing education, practice, and research; experiences the value of practice with clients while mentoring or leading nursing groups; values nursing education by teaching future professionals as well as consuming and contributing to nursing literature; conducts research that substantiates significance of nursing while also acting as consumer of nursing research. Society's image of professional nursing is largely influenced by this level of professional development.

Characteristics of this Stage:

Productive:

- Establishes effective collegial, collaborative, and interpersonal relationships with clients/families/colleagues/coworkers/community

- Facilitates mutual interdisciplinary collaboration and role delegation with client as active partner
- Offers unique contributions to the nursing discipline through organizational leadership, publication of new knowledge gained through professional activities, and regional–national contribution

Nonproductive:

- Competitive for the benefit of self versus the vulnerable client
- Practices in isolation due to lack of collaborative skills and insight into others roles, minimizing impact of care for client
- Health care team experiences nurse as inflexible and dehumanizing

Checking In: To what extent (on a scale of 1-5)

- Do you motivate and guide a group while managing their expectations?
- Do you identify and support the learning needs of individuals, groups and the organization?
- Do you synthesize data from multiple sources to complete a system analysis?
- Do you get the facts before drawing a conclusion?
- Do you listen to another's point of view with an open mind?
- Do you have a powerful and inventive imagination?
- Do you enjoy collaborative adventures with others?

Stage 7—The Older Professional—Focus on Completion
The older professional has opportunities and obligations to complete unfinished business while reflecting on and cherishing their significant contributions and relationships; to offer support and strongly influence the future of nursing through interaction with young professionals, associations and organizations that would benefit from their integrity and their longitudinal perspective on the field.

Characteristics of this Stage:

Productive:

- Derives great personal satisfaction regarding contribution made to the profession and the people served through the years

- Passes on dreams and accomplishments to younger professionals and society
- Experiences pleasure in the achievement of those who follow them

Nonproductive:

- Professional identity marked by a sense of despair
- Cannot recount accomplishments of self or others to celebrate contributions made
- Feels alienation, unsupported and alone

Checking In: To what extent (on a scale of 1–5)

- Do you have a deep sense of faith?
- Do you worry about very little?
- Do you believe that life is not a random event?
- Do you have a sense of contribution from your lifework?
- Do you feel respected and respectful of others?
- Do you enjoy the energy and enthusiasm of youth?
- Do you feel a profound sense of gratitude and peace?

A Living Example

DISCERNING ESSENCE EXERCISE

By focusing on a values cluster profile and sensing into the energy pattern it portrays, you can intuitively perceive the "essence" of any individual or group.

Nursing is a tribe. Within it we have practitioners with interest in one specific aspect of practice. A large values study done on a hospital-based nursing practice revealed that each unit had a distinct profile of the nurses working on that unit. Practice your perceptive skills by studying the five profiles and identifying which group is: Emergency Room, Gerontology, Oncology, Quality Assurance, and Neonatal Intensive Care. Things to consider regarding their work and client population include: the diagnosis of client group, unique needs of the group, inner and outer world focus as it relates to the tasks at hand, amount of autonomy or teamwork required to care for the client population on the unit. Their #1 value is their primary motivator (Figure 6.3).

FIGURE 6.3

Clinical Nursing Group Values Profiles

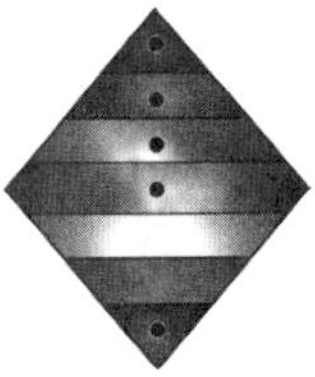

Group #1

TOP Values   Tier Level

1.
2.
3.
4.
5.

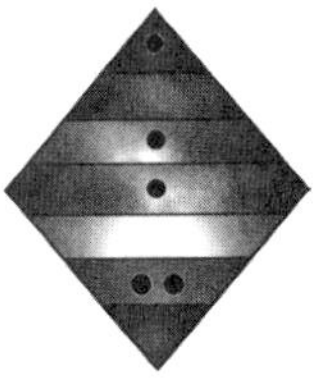

Group #2

TOP Values   Tier Level

1.
2.
3.
4.
5.

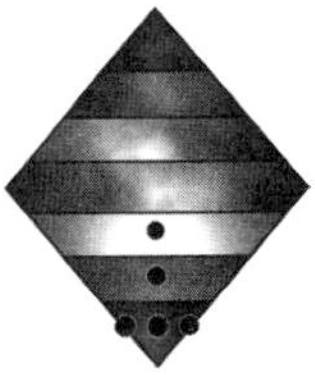

Group #3

TOP Values   Tier Level

1.
2.
3.
4.
5.

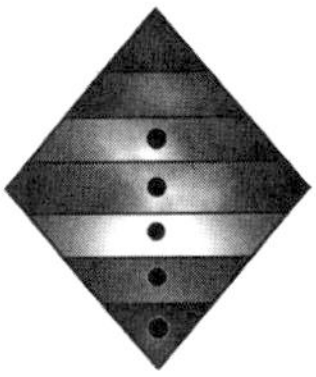

Group #4

TOP Values   Tier Level

1.
2.
3.
4.
5.

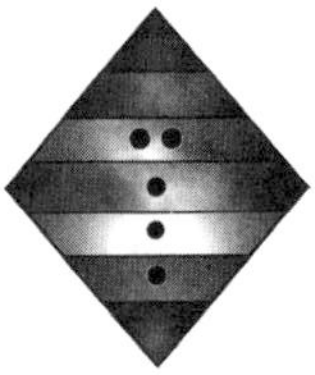

Group #5

TOP Values   Tier Level

1.
2.
3.
4.
5.

Five Slides of Values Profiles

Reflective Questions:

1. Are there common values shared between the groups?
2. What is their style of decision-making?
3. How would the top two values of each group influence their behavior?
4. How would a nurse in Group A fit into the culture of Group C?
5. Identify your top three Professional Values.
6. What behaviors do you manifest that reflect them?
7. What behaviors might you develop further to accentuate them even more?

Web Site Resource: This Web site offers the Values Assessment utilized in this study *http://www.nursemetrix.com*

Answers to the Exercise:

The five leaders in Figure 6.3 are:
A. Gerontology
B. Neonatal Intensive Care
C. Quality Assurance
D. Emergency Room
E. Oncology

BIBLIOGRAPHY

Achterberg, J. (1990). *Woman as healer: A panoramic survey of the healing activities of women from prehistoric times to present.* Boston, MA: Shambhala Press.

Barrett, R. (1998). *Liberating the corporate soul: Building a visionary organization.* Woburn, MA: Butterworth-Heinemann.

Benner, P. (1984). *From novice to expert: Excellence and power in clinical nursing practice.* New York, NY: Springer Publishing Company.

Benner, P., Tanner, C. A., & Chesla, C. A. (1996). *Expertise in nursing practice: Caring, clinical judgment, and ethics.* New York, NY: Springer Publishing Company.

Bodensteiner, L. (2001). Decreasing attrition rates across the generations through values alignment. *Seminar for Nurse Managers, 9*(3), 182–187.

Choquette, S. (2000). *True balance: A commonsense guide for renewing your spirit.* New York, NY: Three Rivers Press.

Coles, R., & Erikson, E. (2000). *The Erik Erikson reader.* New York, NY: WW Norton & Company.

Drucker, P. (1999). *Management challenges for the 21st century.* San Francisco, CA: Harper Collins.

Erikson, E. H. (1980). *Identity and the life cycles.* New York, NY: WW Norton & Company.

Hall, B. P. (1986). *The genesis effect: Personal and organizational transformations.* New York, NY: Paulist Press.

Izzo, J. B., & Withers, P. (1996). *Values shift: The new work ethic & what it means for business.* Toronto, ON: Prentice Hall Canada.

Kumar, S. (2004). The dance of choice and choicelessness. *Shift: At the frontiers of consciousness, 4*(4), 32–35.

Leddy, S., & Pepper, J. M. (1989). *Conceptual bases of professional nursing* (2nd ed.). Philadelphia, PA: JB Lippincott Company.

Lehman, B. (2004). The freedom of yes. *Shift: At the frontiers of consciousness. 4*(4), 11–13.

Leonard, G. (1992). *Mastery: The keys to success and long-term fulfillment.* New York, NY: The Penguin Group.

Lewis, H. (1991). *A question of values: Six ways we make the personal choices that shape our lives.* San Francisco, CA: Harper Collins.

Maslow, A. H. (1980). *The further reaches of human nature.* New York, NY: Penguin Books.

Mezirow, J., & Associates. (1991). *Fostering critical reflection in adulthood: A guide to transformative and emancipatory learning.* San Francisco, CA: Jossey Bass.

Rifkin, J. (2009) *The empathic civilization: The race to global consciousness in a world in crisis.* New York, NY: Penguin Publishing.

Rogers, C. (1980). *A way of being.* New York, NY: Houghton Mifflin.

Thompson, J., & O'Dea, J. (2005). Social healing for a fractured world. *Shift: At the frontiers of consciousness, 7*(3), 10–13.

Thurman, R. (2004). *Infinite life: Seven virtues for living well.* New York, NY: Penguin Group USA.

Chapter 7

Ways of Knowing
Expressions of the Soul

It takes courage to grow up and turn out to be who you really are.

E. E. Cummings

Life is a practical matter. Although theories and scientific proof are important signs and guideposts along the way, every day, in large ways and small, every choice we make creates our life and our reality. We can look out at the world and imagine what it must be like for others, but the only context for living we really understand is our own. The human condition is a complex mixture of messages, experiences, expectations, delights, and limitations, but somewhere deep within, most of us carry an undercurrent of fear. Fear that we are not enough: we don't do enough, we don't know enough, we don't have enough. The personality/ego replays our "best learned messages" over and over again in endless succession until we become what our mind chatter tells us.

The sad truth is that within that same amazing mind lies another story that is the real truth: we are, each one of us, authentic, amazing, gifted, and blessed with capacity and opportunity as we recognize what is right in front of us. While life circumstance and physical and mental capacity varies, within each of us lies a deeper way of knowing and being in the world. The outer world of ego personality is programmed and scripted in mindless fashion. When we shift our focus to the inner world of own unique soul guided by our Spiritual Ego, a new world opens. Living from this larger truth is the doorway to freedom, peace, and love.

All of us want to affect the world for the better. America is a society of rules. We look around at the problems of crime, drug abuse, child neglect—and congress enacts laws to correct them.

Ancient Greece, on the other hand, was a culture of ideas and concepts. Verbal exchange between great minds such as Socrates and Aristotle gave birth to dialogue as a creative examination of idea. This led to the emergence of philosophy as a new, expansive way of viewing reality and responding to it. Laws restrict and maintain, whereas fresh ideas expand and transcend. Balance between the two is the hallmark of wisdom.

In contrast, Native American culture assumes that if something is to be changed it requires a shift in perception. Rather than making laws or creating new theories, they choose to change the way they see the problem. By shifting their focus they change a challenge into an opportunity. In this way, they dream their world into being (Villoldo, 2006, 2010).

We are living on the edge of a new era where a shift in conscious awareness is moving us beyond thinking and ego personality into the deeper world of our Spiritual Ego in touch with Universal Wisdom and the Inner Wisdom of our soul. Presence is the individual manifestation of our stage on this "Soul Journey." It is not something we can "do or learn." Rather, it is something we simply are—*our way of being*—which is felt by others. Vibrational essence is the hallmark of consciousness. It is the spiritual fabric and moral imperative that impels us forward.

Little children are completely authentic, with actions guided by instinct and emotions. They listen to the silent promptings of their own integrity from a framework of wholeness. They gather *information* from multiple sources both formal and exploratory in nature. As they learn to navigate the world and engage in shared relationships through thought, word, and action, their attention gets programmed with *knowledge;* concepts, rules, assumptions, and beliefs. Slowly, simple awareness is replaced with an incessant stream of assumptions and thoughts.

As our attention gets increasingly focused on the information and knowledge in our heads and the predominant mass culture, we no longer perceive the world through the eyes of innocence and unconditional love. We see only that which we have learned to believe, missing the true presence of Inner Wisdom. The analytic voice of information and knowledge never stops talking, judging, gossiping, and filling our life with background noise and distraction. It sabotages our happiness and keeps us from enjoying the reality of authenticity, truth, and love in the moment. This too, is a stage of development.

The path to *wisdom* is an ongoing movement from the innocence of childhood, through the years of information and knowledge acquisition and management, ever evolving toward increased understanding and higher intelligence. Wisdom—a shift in focus—is a return to the stage of wonder. However, this time we possess a discernment distilled from our lived experience, which turns borrowed knowledge into our own truth. Life once again becomes an expression of our authentic self with a knowing that transcends articulation.

Occasionally, we come in contact with something that defies understanding; a moment of *mystery*. When we stand in the presence of the Unknowable, we are filled with a sense of awe, wonder, and an illumined knowing that transcends thought. In that moment, we are standing on sacred ground, a space pulsating with a disclosure of the Universal Truth.

While our outer purpose is to grow and change over time, our inner purpose is to remember the truth of who we are. Instead of being lost in thinking, we recognize ourselves as the awareness behind the thought. Awareness takes charge from the thinking that has governed our lives and connects us with our true soul. A shift in focus occurs from outer to inner authority, and we begin to live from the vantage point of higher mind, home of our Spiritual Ego.

Teilhard de Chardin suggests we need a "lookout point in the universe" as we launch into the next phase of human evolution. Peaceful existence cannot rely on thinking or reason; we must follow a deeper organic rhythm. In the center of our soul lies our "Inner Wisdom," which will lovingly guide us into each tomorrow as we uncover and manifest the inner voice that is ours.

Self-remembering is the "soul's journey," the way we use life experiences to grow and deepen as human beings. Moving through the various "ways of knowing" until we arrive in close communion with our own "Inner Wisdom" evolves as we practice the art of remembering. In her compelling book, *Standing Stark*, conscious living teacher Carla Woody guides us in ways to live an unencumbered life (2004). She suggests that what we hold inside our minds as true and possible forms the edge of our reality. Building on the path breaking work of mythologist Joseph Campbell, she presents the "transformational" remembering process in five stages (pp. 171–178):

1. *Sparking* is the awakening from an unconscious life, usually slowly and over a period of time. The task is to wake up to the current state of our lives.
2. *Separation* is a time of unlearning and uncoupling. Examination of jobs, relationships, homes, and beliefs; nothing is exempt from this in-depth sorting and releasing.
3. *Searching* leads to widening choices. Increasingly we explore areas that are new and different, discovering what fits our core SELF.
4. *Initiation* is the process of assimilation of our increased awareness and new ways of "being" into our lives. We drop all masks and pretense, appreciate the old life for all its gifts, and step beyond with intent.
5. *Re-entry* calls us to immersion back into the world in which we live. We are now ready to share, teach, support, and guide others undertaking a similar journey.

As we being to live with the clarity that emerges as outworn patterns are cast aside, we start to move with the energetic rhythms of the Universe, experiencing ever-increasing cycles of flow and synchronicity.

SHIFTING FOCUS—A LIFE EXAMINED

When we bring our attention to the inner world of soul, struggle ceases. The first thing to change is our perspective, and this will change the way our life unfolds. A shift in focus is a mini-breakthrough in awareness—it is a moment of In-Sight! One small piece of conditioned thinking is shattered. Instead of being victim to a rigid belief, we feel empowered as the trapped energy is released. We become more fluid, flexible, open and creative. This occurs as our attention moves toward the soul, the unprogrammed part of ourselves. The soul never says no, for everything is possible in this field of unlimited potential. As we being to live from the perspective of our higher mind, every day is a series of In-Sight! moments that guide our decisions in the direction of our destiny.

To enhance our consciousness through release of outmoded patterns of thought and behavior, awareness must guide us. We must catch ourselves in the act of "thinking." We must become aware of the countless little rules, assumptions and expectations that keep saying "no" before we are even aware that there might be other ways of viewing a situation. Practices in mindfulness that prompt In-Sight! are the hallmark of a postmodern nurse.

We can only learn so many lessons alone. It is the nature of all cells and species to find strength and wisdom in community. Others who have gone before us have left guideposts for our journey from innocence and information to wisdom and wholeness. In their own way, each has observed that *expanding personal awareness is the key to wholeness.*

Translation of experience into words, metaphors and stories allows us to share the insight gleaned by others. The following is a collection of observations expressed by patients, professionals, and family care givers alike. Their role has not been identified because you will see the universal nature of their articulated wisdom. Focusing questions and growth opportunities are also offered as a guide to further developing your In-Sight!

In a true healing relationship, both heal and both are healed.

Rachel Naomi Remen

I—INFORMATION: THE WORLD AS MIRROR OF THE MIND

It is important to understand that the science and logic we call reality is a manifestation of the world our mind creates, a reflection of our beliefs and our intentions.

Focusing Questions for Conscious Living—Living the Examined Life

Why do you do what you do? What is your intention for helping?

In truth, no one had ever adequately prepared me for the wonders of [caregiving]: the emotional ups and downs; the spiritual element that can tax one's faith, can shake it to its very foundation;

the observation of miracles; and the growth and development that occur beyond one's wildest imagination. In the final analysis, nursing puts us in touch with being human.

M. Patricia Donahue

I served for many dysfunctional reasons. I served so that you would like me. I became a nurse so that I could look at your problems instead of my own. I served so that I could feel in control. When not in control, I felt an inner anxiety that stemmed from an uncontrollable past. I served so that I could feel needed, since I needed to be needed. I served so that you would give me esteem, because I could not give myself any.

Caryn Summers

We sometimes speak as if caring did not require knowledge, as if caring for someone, for example, were simply a matter of good intentions or warm regard. But in order to care I must understand the other's needs and I must be able to respond properly to them, and clearly good intentions do not guarantee this. I do not try to help the other grow in order to actualize myself, but by helping the other grow I do actualize myself.

Milton Mayeroff

I came to [caregiving] without my own thinking; using research or others' ideas as my own, feeling ashamed of thoughts I had about healing, and fearful, believing I didn't have the right to speak up or out. Unaware of my neediness, I was able to use the theories of others and take care of others to shore myself up. I excelled, and my colleagues fed me the definition of myself that I created for them. I never felt full.

David Willard

What is true healing? And what is the place of the healer within the healing process? In my eighty years, I seemed to experiment with a whole range of answers to these vital questions. Through the process of "discovering the healer," with its leaps of understanding and moments of self-discovery, I have experienced the vital importance of a surrendered heart. When our primary motivation is to be totally available to the life process, any distinction between "healer" and "healee" disappears, and there is only one I AM.

Frances Horn

It is important to gain self/other knowledge as part of spiritual growth and balance—to know yourself and believe in yourself means you can know and believe in God. Knowledge of yourself produces humility, and knowledge of God produces love.

Mother Teresa

Sad that so often [helping] imprisons us, that because of it we find ourselves accomplices to conditions of separateness and division—a world of nurses and patients, social workers and clients, spiritual teachers and seekers, people who know and people who don't. After all, if some of us are busy being helpers there must be others under continuous pressure to be helped. If I stop to think about it, I help out for all kinds of reasons. Maybe it's because I should; it's a matter of responsibility. But there's usually a maze of other motives: a need for self-esteem, approval, status, power; the desire to feel useful, find intimacy, and pay back some debt.

Ram Dass

With modernization, changing social norms create the need to critically examine the paradigms of thought which we were taught by dominant culture to understand our experience. The process of self-reflection has the potential for profoundly changing the way we make sense of the world, other people and ourselves. Transformative learning, in turn, leads to actions that significantly change the character of our interpersonal relationships, the organizations we work in and socialize, and the world itself.

Jack Mezirow

Growth Opportunity

Cultivate self-knowledge through the process of reflection. *Reflection in action* requires focused awareness in the moment. One acts reflexively as well as reflectively as the unique needs of the patient are considered along with the scripts of standardization. *Reflection on action* involves a purposeful review of a significant event after it is over, examining of one's own motives and actions along with their impact on the situation and its outcome.

Focusing Questions for Vibrant Health—
Being the Change You Want to See in the World

What is your definition of health? How do you manage and model your health beliefs?

Self-care cannot be accomplished without self-love. We need to ask if we feel worthy enough to care for ourselves, even as a priority over caring for others. We are most effective as caregivers when we are centered in our own sense of well-being.

Caryn Summers

For so much of my life I was run by this nagging voice in the back of my head that kept saying, "You're not doing enough! You're not doing enough!" But now I'm starting to listen to my body a lot more. It needs tender loving care and I'm the only one who can provide that. Even though I always feared that if I took better care of myself it would mean I'd become selfish or self indulgent, I've discovered that's not the case.

Leonard Felder

Some things in life can not be avoided: death, illness, change, personal expectations. What each of them does to us depends a great deal on the way we have allowed ourselves to deal with lesser things. Stability centers us in something greater than ourselves so that nothing lesser than ourselves can possibly sweep us away.

Joan Chittister

When experiencing difficulty in discerning your own needs, it may be helpful to begin by observing what you provide for others. Often we give to other people what we unconsciously know that we need ourselves.

Carmen Renee Berry

Beyond treating the symptom, the physician has the responsibility representing wellness to the patient, of being a totem of wellness rather than a figure associated only with disease.

Dawson Church

To love yourself is to heal yourself.

Course in Miracles

Health is not equivalent to happiness, surfeit, or success. It is fore-most a matter of being wholly one with whatever circumstances we find ourselves in. Even our death is a healthy event if we fully embrace the fact of our dying....The issue is awareness, of living in the present. Whatever our present existence consists of, if we are at one with it, we are healthy.

Elizabeth Kubler-Ross

If I don't do me, I don't get done.

Jacquelyn Small

Every day is another chance to discover more about yourself—what are your strengths and limitations as a caregiver; what are you really like as a family member or friend; what are you learning about your own ability to express love, patience, and caring; and what are you discovering about your priorities in life?

Leonard Felder

Growth Opportunity

Cultivate healthy balance in your life. Identifying and managing your personal issues are as critical to vibrant health as diet and nutrition...it is an on-going process of discovery, forgiveness and release. Pay attention to little tugs and resistances and discern when you felt like that before. What is it stirring up for you? How can you bless it, transcend it, and move on?

Focusing Questions for Focused Clarity— Seeing the Whole Rather than the Hole

What is your personal accountability in any situation, in your life, to all of life?

Our most profound growth comes during our most painful times. Becoming aware of the difficulty is the first step in finding the solution. Once we acknowledge our despair and admit that we are powerless, we become empowered. Once we admit that our lives are unmanageable, we no longer have to pretend to be in control. By stating our confusion, we make the first move toward clarity. When denial stops, the process of healing begins. In the center of chaos lies the promise of clarity.

Caryn Summers

The best gift a serious illness gives us is the ability to become "clear"…to accept our troubled areas-fear, doubt, and love ourselves in spite of them. The best gift you can give yourself and others is the gift of clarity. It takes fear, doubt, etc. and makes them disappear. Go inside to uncover the hidden mysteries of your self and then jump on the outside to see how your "healing" can begin the "healing" for someone else. GET CLEAR! I would rather be clear for 1 day then to live to be 100 in the dark. The gift I would give myself would outlive me because it would change the consciousness of those I love most. That is one of the most significant purposes of living and we often don't even see it. Illness can be the ultimate gift if you surrender, embrace and love all that it brings into your life for better or worse…because you see their never has been or will be a worse. When you get clear on this all else will be just as it should.

Kristi Welch

Its more about living life well than keeping the law perfectly…. It involves a conscious gathering of the wisdom of others who can encourage us and help us scrutinize our own choices for their value and their valor. Learn to see what you are looking at and then say what you see. Looking is so difficult in our culture which is highly technological and intent on fixing on what is not broken.

Joan Chittister

What is to give light must endure burning.

Vicktor Frankl

I have a clear choice between life and death, between reality and fantasy, between health and sickness. I have to become responsible— responsible for mistakes as well as accomplishments.

Eileen Mayhew

We labor under the myth that it is the ministrations of healthcare providers that cure or heal people. This is simply an illusion, a product of faulty logic. The assumption is that if a patient gets well after surgery, she gets well because of surgery. The reality is that surgery does not cure/heal. Drugs do not cure/heal. Acupuncture, or crystals, or homeopathy do not cure/heal. The person who undergoes the surgery, or takes the drug, or receives the alternative treatment must heal herself. Any or all of the above-named ministrations may be necessary to removed barriers to self-healing or to stimulate it, but they are not sufficient causes for healing.

Janet F. Quinn

Have the courage to act instead of react.

Darlene Larson Jenks

Being stuck in the past is just another form illusion can take. The message seems to be: Complete, with honesty, whatever is bothering you, and then…stop looking back.

Jacquelyn Small

Life is tragic, but not necessarily serious. We are small people, here for a while. The sounds will soon cover over our seemingly important enterprises. Let's do our best, respect each other, and hope that someone's passage is the better for our existence.

John Neil

Growth Opportunity

A choice point exists where past and future overlap. Cultivate your decision-making capacity without wearing dark or rose colored glasses. Release fears created in past experiences and expectations for future outcomes. Let the moment guide your course of action by seeing it for what it is and trusting the process of life toward greater good.

II—KNOWLEDGE: LIVED EXPERIENCE AS TEACHER

I may have misinformation, but I never have a misexperience.

De Lorian

Focusing Questions for Reverence for Life—
Holding an Interconnected View of the Universe

What comprises your world view? How are things related and how do they work?

Each thing on earth holds a spark of life. Seeing and appreciating its beauty is the recognition of our shared spark from the creator. All things are our relatives.

Wanigi Waci

For me there is a reverence for life. It means enjoying the sunshine, the rain, a dust storm, walking down the city street, and looking to see the pleasure, to smell the fresh air. It means bringing the country with me to the city. It's working hard in my garden. It's reading a good book. It's being with people I enjoy. It's even being with people I don't enjoy. It's learning to choose. It's learning I can't care for everyone. It's having an obligation not to cause pain in this life and to ease it when I can.

Nola Pennert

Alone I am what I am, but in community I have the chance to become everything that I can be. Humility is a basic awareness of my relationship to the world and my connectedness to all its circumstances....There is no haughtiness, distance, sarcasm, put downs, airs of importance or disdain. The ability to deal with our own and others limitations flows from the recognition that God is in life, relieving us from being in charge of the universe. This brings serenity and hope, inner peace and energy.

Joan Chittister

There is in every true heart a spark of heavenly fire, Which lies dormant in the broad daylight of prosperity; But which kindles up and beams and blazes In the dark hour of adversity.

Anonymous Proverb

We are healed of a suffering only by experiencing it to the full.

Marcel Proust

To understand ourselves and our place in the world, we might pay more attention to the natural laws, to the life cycle of animals and plants. Nature reflects the Universal Laws. Oversee its working in the habits of birds, the cycles of plants, and the instincts of reptiles and mammals. All teach the secrets of life. Watch the coming and going of clouds, the waxing and waning of the moon, the rising and setting of the sun. They reveal the natural order of creation. Everything is right when there is neither too much nor too little for the time and place.

Harold Klemp

Loving others is an expression of our love for God.

Mother Teresa

I ask, how would nature solve this? I try to think like nature to find the right questions. You don't invent answers; you reveal the answers from nature. In nature the answers to all our problems already exist.

Dr. Jonas Salk

When we learn both to take and to give, we can move into a flow of giving and receiving that is love's essence—reciprocity. In this way, the flow of energy does not go just one way, but both. I give to you and you to me and we both fully receive the energy. Christ said to "love your neighbor as yourself." Sacrifice, how-ever, has been misinterpreted as loving your neighbor instead of yourself.

Carol S Pearson

The fragrance of the rose lingers on the hand of the giver.

Unknown Teacher

Growth Opportunity

Cultivate an appreciation for beauty in music, the arts, and nature. Explore the new discoveries in space, quantum science, and technology as well as economics, social sciences and spirituality. Become informed about environmental issues, and practice a sim-plistic lifestyle of "living lightly on the earth."

What is your life story? How does it enrich and limit your continuing unfolding?

When one is a stranger to oneself, then one is estranged from others.... if one is out of touch with oneself, then one cannot touch others.

Anne Morrow Lindbergh

Authentic service can be seen in the nurse who has nurtured herself, the healer who has been healed. It is the service we hear when the nurse can speak from her heart to the patient these simply and humble words, "I am here". Let's heal together."

Caryn Summers

Life is lived in cycles of seven years. Every seven years all cells are replaced in your body, and they are genetically influenced by your ancestors. What happens in your life emotionally and spiritually also touches seven generations. As the middle [forth] generation, your influence extends from you back to your parents, your grandparents and great-grandparents. It also goes out from you to your child, grand children and great-grandchildren. Healing efforts made on your part will also heal them, while injuries you create will also hurt them. Remember the accountability you have to seven generations each time you make a decision.

Wanigi Waci

First try to discover your own childhood, then take the experience seriously....Try to feel, and help the patient to feel....study the history of childhood....Therapy has to open you as well as the patient for feeling in your life. It has to awaken you from a sleep.

Alice Miller

The most elusive knowledge of all is self-knowledge.

Mirra Komarovsky

When you look upon another and feel great love towards them, or when you contemplate beauty in nature and something within you responds deeply, close your eyes for a moment and feel the essence of that love or beauty, inseparable from who you are, your true nature. The outer form is a temporary reflection of what you are within, in your essence. That is why love and beauty can never leave you, although all outer forms will.

Eckhart Tolle

To me, healing is releasing from the past. It is retraining my mind so as not to see the shadow of the past on anyone. It is learning not to make interpretations of people's behavior or motives. It is letting go of the desire to want to change another person. It is letting go of expectations, assumptions, and the desire to control or manipulate another person.

Gerald Tampolsky

The curriculum of service provides us with information about our strengths and our weaknesses; we discover how these contribute to genuinely help-full service. Each time we drop our masks and meet heart-to-heart, reassuring one another simply by the quality of our presence, we experience a profound bond which we intuitively understand is nourishing everyone.

Ram Dass

What we grew up with, we learned;
What we learned, we practiced;
And what we practiced, we became.

Ernie Larsen

Growth Opportunity

Become familiar with your life story. Know your own attitudes, values, and beliefs so that you do not project them onto others. Visit friends and relatives to get other perspectives. Know your family of origin, and recognize the patterns you inherited. Purposefully choose which ones to maintain and which to forgive and transcend. Be the example you want your children to become.

Focusing Questions for Creative Imagination—
Shedding outworn beliefs and expectations

What rules govern your reality? How do you transcend them?

Healing in the future must involve major shifts in the way we think about health and illness. The focus of a health-care system must be on facilitating wholeness, which means facilitating right relationship. The techniques are beside the point. What must occur is twofold: the revaluing of the feminine principle and its ways, and the empowerment of individuals and communities to create their own health and healing.

Janet Quinn

Life is either a daring adventure or nothing.

Helen Keller

It is time to break free of our overly serious approach to life and laugh, have fun, cultivate frivolity and joy. We [helpers] need to learn how to say "Yes!"—to having fun, to going on adventures, to attending spiritual retreats, to spontaneous outings, to developing our artistic talents, to listening to music, to reading enjoyable books, to soaking in bubble baths, to exercising regularly, to filling our homes with cut flowers and beauty and art.

Carmen Renee Berry

Every atom is striving continually to manifest more life; all are intelligent, and all are seeking to carry out the purpose for which they were created. Life is a mystery until we begin to understand that we can be the creators of our own world and that, in truth, what we are today is a creation of that which we have made from the past.

Paul Twitchell

Artistic creation, sports, dance, teaching, counseling—mastery in any field of endeavor implies that the thinking mind is either no longer involved at all or at least is taking second place. A power and intelligence greater than you and yet one with you in essence takes over. There is no decision-making process anymore; spontaneous right action happens...Mastery of life is the opposite of control. You become aligned with the greater consciousness. It acts, speaks, does the work.

Eckhart Tolle

Only those who dare truly live.

Ruth P. Freedman

Develop a sense of humor, and as challenges come up, you begin to draw on your creativity. You find solutions that would never have occurred to you before. Life becomes more fun—you have a more adventuresome life. You get put into situations you would not have been in before, because you are going one step beyond yourself. And as you get yourself in trouble, you also have help to get out of it, because as you learn to work with your own resources, you are developing self-mastery.

Harold Klemp

Take two jokes and call me in the morning.

Unknown Teacher

Thought creates form, but it is feeling that gives vitality to the thought.

Unknown Teacher

Growth Opportunity

Transcend the silent rules and assumptions that govern your reality by observing nature and young children at play. Reclaim your birthright: a deep sense of awe, wonder and discovery fostered by non-ego dominated exploration. Refine the ability to identify thought patterns blocked and stunted by desire or intellect. Open space for spontaneous creation to emerge by increasing your ability to see potential and possibility in every situation rather than stopping at a scripted standard.

III—WISDOM: PRESENT MOMENT AS GUIDE

Wisdom is not a product of thought. The deep knowing that is wisdom arises through the simple act of giving someone your full attention. Attention is primordial intelligence.

Eckhart Tolle

**Focusing Questions for Courageous Vigilance—
Bearing Witness to Suffering With Mercy-Full Detachment**

What is hard for you to look at or acknowledge? How do you determine and establish boundaries in an encounter?

Detachment doesn't mean not to get involved; it means to not let outer circumstances throw off your inner balance. We will all have a certain amount of pain and pleasure, but will not let it overly affect our emotional balance if we are detached from fear. Only when fear is in control of those two poles is your life attached to its physical, mental and spiritual possessions. Give up fear and you need never give up another thing in your life. Great joys can become yours, balanced by what sorrows need to be in your life.

Harold Klemp

Those who do not know how to weep with their whole heart don't know how to laugh either.

Goldia Meir

Unless we as healers are willing to confront our own pain and darkness, we can never be truly open to that joining of energy with our patients that is necessary for the fullest healing process to take place for both.

Niravni Payne

The abuse of power is solving problems for people that belong to them.

Stewart Block

No excuse is good enough for neglecting to reach out and embrace our loved ones while they are still alive. Death can come when we least expect it, so we must take every opportunity to give our love [and presence] to those around us. The time is now!

Barry and Joyce Vissell

To detach means to give others the freedom to grow through their own mistakes and experiences. It is not feeling responsible for others, but rather allowing others to learn self-responsibility.

Caryn Summers

You heal a brother by recognizing his worth.

Course in Miracles

To study the Way is to study the Self.
To study the Self is to forget the Self.
To forget the Self is to be enlightened by all things.
To be enlightened by all things is to remove the barrier
Between Self and Other.

Dogen Zenji

Trust in the other to grow and in my own ability to care gives me courage to go into the unknown, but it is also true that without the courage to go in the unknown such trust would be impossible.

Milton Mayeroff

Courage is the price that life extracts for peace. Courage is the last uncrowded place in the Universe.

Amelia Erhart

Growth Opportunity

Cultivate your dark side. Until there is self-awareness, unconscious projection and roll-playing makes up a large part of human inter-action. By letting go of your resistance to the hard things in life, you become vulnerable. This softens the hard and rigid parts of your soul, making you available to yourSelf and others. By being at risk, you will discover and share your true essential nature, which is the same essence in all of humanity.

Focusing Questions for Elegant Timing— Practicing Effortless Learning and Living

---

What prompts you to act? How much effort is expended for the outcome obtained?

There have been great leaders such as Lincoln and King across history. While there have been many able men, at certain times the personality, the needs and values of society align in such a way that the individual is literally propelled into a leadership position. Timing is the essence of wisdom. If it is too difficult, and you find yourself pulling or pushing, the time is not right. Patience and dis-cernment are the antidotes to poor timing.

Emil Erikson

Each person faces a time of danger and a time of potential transfor-mation. It's not for any of us to judge their response. It is for us to "be there" for them, not necessarily to "do" for them.

Rraeme Amontee

You must be careful to do what is appropriate and evolutionary for the other. Otherwise you become a compulsive cornucopia, burying someone under all the gifts you are pouring out. Your apparent gen-erosity is not always appreciated, and indeed maybe deeply resented.

Jean Houston

An easy litmus test can determine whether one is giving or enabling. If, when we give, we feel either used or smugly superior; it is time to look at what really is going on. Healthy giving is respectful of both the giver and the receiver.

Carol S. Pearson

There is a divine plan of good at work in my life. I will let go and let it unfold.

Ruth P. Freedman

Effortless learning and effortless living occurs when you quit striving. As a Harvard student I applied myself but got mediocre grades. One huge college assignment was given in comparative literature. I put it off because of its difficulty until the night before it was due. Rather than reading the thick volumes of Freud and Durkheim, I literally skimmed through the books, underlining anything that leaped out as interesting. I began to notice that here and there some of their ideas were opposed or in alignment. I marked those places and typed whatever came to me about the two. I had no choice; I had to do it. It was interesting and fun to write. I was relaxed, enjoying it because I knew I was going to get an F. That paper was the first and only A+ that I ever got at Harvard.

Gary Zukav

Care-giving and rescuing are a lot different. Rescuing can make the rescuer feel good; but it might not make the patient feel good.

Dave Morris

I slept and dreamt that life was joy,
I awoke and saw that life was service,
I acted and behold, service was joy.

Rabindranath Tagore

There is a thin line between giving and unhealthy "enabling" (i.e., supporting someone else's dependency or irresponsibility). Sometimes we persist in giving to people who use our gifts and energy only to help themselves continue in a destructive pattern.

Carlos Petres

Growth Opportunity

Cultivate the capacity to identify the subtle in all things. Intuition is the recognition of pattern by sensing slight shifts leading toward disruption. Develop trust in your own wisdom in-the-moment and respond in real time instead of waiting for affirmation from external "experts." Be present in the "now" for it holds all the information needed for right timing.

Focusing Questions for Compassionate Caring— Expressing Nonjudgment and Forgiveness for All

How do you demonstrate caring to others, to yourself?
What problems are yours to solve?

Nothing may be more important than being gentle with ourselves. Whether we're professionals working a sixty-hour week or simply family members called upon to care daily for a sick relative, facing suffering continuously is no small task. We learn the value of recognizing our limits, forgiving ourselves our bouts of impatience or guilt, acknowledging our own needs. We see that to have compassion for others we must have compassion for ourselves.

Ram Dass

Caring for others is a deepening process. We begin with sympathy; "I feel sorry for you." It is an act of separation for you are experiencing something I am not. Then comes the state of empathy; "I am one with you, I can relate." In this space we find our similarity and shared connection. This is followed by a mature state of compassion; "I am distressed for you, myself and all who are in a similar state, including the earth". Here we are at-one with the world, and the depth of our emotion compels us to social action—to correct the injustice against all beings.

Matthew Fox

It is not how much you do but how much love you put into the doing and sharing with others that is important. Try not to judge people. If you judge others then you are not giving love.

Mother Teresa

As our understanding of our own suffering deepens, we become available at deeper levels to those we would care for. We are less likely to project suffering that does not exist or deny that which does. We're much more sensitive and alert to the nuances of human pain. Compassion and pity are very different. Whereas compassion reflects the yearning of the heart to merge and take on some of the suffering, pity is a controlled set of thoughts designed to assure separateness. Compassion is the spontaneous response of life, pity, the involuntary reflex of fear.

Ram Dass

When we see another person with problems, we can have compassion; but we understand that somewhere down the path these problems have emerged by his own efforts. While we can offer compassion and support, we must let him have the freedom to experience his troubles. People of good intentions—who are often short on patience—sometimes forget the Law of Non-interference.

Harold Klemp

All the healing techniques in the world won't really help unless love goes with them.

Louise L. Hay

Caring is the antithesis of simply using the other person to satisfy one's own needs.

Milton Mayeroff

No one ever becomes a perfect being. There is always one more step towards wholeness. We always seek, but never find, completion.

Harold Klemp

Growth Opportunity

Cultivate the capacity for nonjudgment and forgiveness of yourself and others. As you surrender the striving for perfection, you quit putting impossible demands on every situation, person, place, or event. Your life, and the experience of others whom you touch, becomes more harmonious and peaceful. A state of "nonresistance" opens you to universal awareness which is vastly greater than your human mind. You move naturally with the flow and timing of events, enriched by respect for the resilience of the human spirit and the divine.

IV—MYSTERY: THE UNKNOWN AS INSPIRATION

Become at ease with the state of "not knowing." This takes you beyond the mind which is always trying to conclude and interpret... Truth is far more all-encompassing than mind could ever comprehend.

Eckhart Tolle

**Focusing Questions for Learned Ignorance—
Releasing the Need for Certainty and Predictability**

---

*How do you discern the lesson offered in each situation?
What memory or belief may be released or reframed?*

An attitude of not having anything further to learn is incompatible with caring.

Milton Mayeroff

The reward, the real grace of conscious service....is the opportunity not only to help relieve suffering but to grow in wisdom, experience greater unity, and have a good time while we're doing it.

Ram Dass

I don't think we can stand back and look at ourselves and our culture and the way we live in the world, raping the world, without feeling sad. I try to see life like a lake. The anger and the politics and the bitching and the back-biting and essence of humanizing comes from the deep, dark blue waters underneath. That's where the dolphins and the whales swim. That's where the mysteries are.

Graeme Greer

The body knows and the soul knows: only our minds can lie.

Jacquelyn Small

Being a good teacher requires a willingness to take the risk of inviting open dialogue, knowing I can never predict where it is going to take us. I can then see my student's life more clearly than they do, opening a capacity to look beyond their initial self-presentation, helping them see themselves more clearly.

Parker Palmer

The longer I practice medicine, the less sure I am of the dividing line between healer and those in need of healing. Patients whose overwhelming physical problems made me feel useless have taught me volumes about the true nature of my calling, thereby restoring my faith in myself as a doctor.

Bernie Siegel

The harder a person struggles to achieve some goal, the more difficulty he will have to overcome; difficulty caused at least in part, by the strain of his effort. When your attention leaves your mind and moves into the Now, there is an alertness....Such clarity, such simplicity. No room for problem-making. Just this moment as it is.

Eckhard Tolle

One cannot have wisdom without living life.

Dorothy McCall

I have learned to stand back and let the divine work through me. It is facilitated by adopting a certain attitude of curious, childlike devotion. Many people seek this state but the urgency of their physical needs causes tension and fear, closing the channel between themselves and the Spirit. Competition intensifies the attitude of tension; tensions springs from fear; fear rises out of excessive self-love; excessive self-love cuts one off from the qualities leading to satisfaction, happiness, new insights and growth.

Lai Tsi

We each choose our own state of conscious knowing. We make our own worlds. Life carries all people and beings onward to the expansion of consciousness. Across our lifespan, through the use of experience and reflection on that experience, we move from innocence to disillusionment, and then on to conscious innocence.

Phyllis Jones

Growth Opportunity

Cultivate the capacity for humility. Recognize that we do not always know or have the answers. Release the need for certainty and predictability, reveling in the true wonder of the moment. Develop an ability to trust and move forward even, especially, when we do not know the "how" or "why" of a situation or opportunity. Recognizing and acknowledging what we do not know is the beginning of freedom.

Focusing Questions for Active Surrender— Utilizing the Power of Paradox

What opposing energies are present in this situation?
Where is the middle ground?

We must want to be human as well as efficient; to be loving as well as informed; to be caring as well as knowledgeable; to be happy as well as respected. Attendant listening and watching teaches us critical discernment; it evaluates everything, not in the light of what is good for me, but in the light of what is best for all of us. It brings us to growth, to truth and the holy responsibility for the lives of the entire human community.

Joan Chittister

You must learn to be still in the midst of activity and to be vibrantly alive in repose.

Indira Gandhi

Here in the intensive neonatal care unit you see the incredible beauty and the unbearable pain. And you have to figure out how to be with both.

A Nurse

It was in the darkness that I found the light. It was in the pain that I found the gain. It was in the dying that I found the life. It was in the aloneness that I found the need of prayer. And it is through the love of God that I found meaning in my life.

A Patient

Never try to force results. The more you try to put your imaginative powers upon something in concentrated effort, the less you can do it. Outcome is concerned with imagining and feeling. What you image you must feel—therefore the negative impact of striving is more likely to be effective than vivid imagining because the negative has strong feeling with it.

Harold Klemp

The woundedness in each of us connects us in trust. My woundedness evokes your healer, and your woundedness evokes my healer. Then the two healers can collaborate together.

Rachel Naomi Remen

The reason you cannot earn your worth is because you are already worthy. All you can do is accept what is already yours.

Carmen Renee Berry

The beauty of the world has two edges, one of laughter, one of anguish, cutting the heart asunder.

Virginia Woolf

Wounding is the traditional training ground for the healer. Those who have, through accident or illness, vividly confronted the reality of their own death often return to life with a renewed sense of wonder and strength.

Jean Houston

True selflessness is not the abandonment of self, but rather the surrender of selfish motives. The result of this surrender is self love, or self-esteem. We experience our preciousness and value and reach out from that centered place of love, serving authentically.

Caryn Summers

Growth Opportunity

Bring balance to complex situations by utilizing the power of paradox. Cultivate the ability to "simply be" with an event, releasing the need for control. With your intuitive presence identify the polarities and seek the point of connection where the passive middle lies. Here is the point of reconciliation, the space from which new order will emerge and form.

Focusing Questions for Mindful Awareness— Stepping Beyond Mind into the "Moment" With Fresh Eyes

What do you "hear" when you listen with your inner ear? What do you "see" when you look through eyes of discernment?

The equivalent of external noise is the inner noise of thinking. The equivalent of external silence is inner stillness. But what is wisdom, and where is it to be found? Wisdom comes with the ability to be still. Just look and just listen. No more is needed. Being still, looking, and listening activates the non-conceptual intelligence within you. Let stillness direct your words and actions.

Eckhart Tolle

The heart does speak most eloquently if we listen with our inner ear. Nursing reaches out to the hearts of others to assist as midwives in the birthing of new consciousness. Nurses have frequent opportunities to facilitate the transformation of the experience of discomfort and disease into one of growth, renewal and opportunity. Let the heart speak clearly, and it will touch the world around!

Susanne Davis

When we learn to be where we are, we gain perspective on life. Yesterday loses its hold on us and tomorrow loses its allure.... Mindfulness makes the present, and gives us back the energy that endless worry and constant calculation drain. It concentrates what has become scattered and brings us home to ourselves.

Joan Chittister

If we are willing to examine the agitation of our own minds and look just beyond it, we quite readily find entry into rooms that hold surprising possibilities: a greater inner calm, sharper concentration, deeper intuitive understanding, and an enhanced ability to hear one another's heart. Such an inquiry turns out to be critical in the work of helping others.

Ram Dass

Learn to get in touch with silence within yourself and know that everything in this life has a purpose. There are no mistakes, no coincidences. All events are blessings given to us to learn from.

Elizabeth Kubler-Ross

People who cannot live comfortably with silence can never live comfortably with noise. Silence and inactivity is a frightening thing: it leaves us at the mercy of the noise within. Silence invites us to depth...it heals what hoarding and running will not touch.

Joan Chittister

The longest journey is the journey inward, for he who has chosen his destiny has started upon his quest for the source of his being.

Dag Hammarsjkold

When you meet anyone, remember it is a holy encounter. Thoughtfulness, the kindly regard for others, is the beginning of holiness.

Mother Teresa

When the higher incorporates the lower into its service, the nature of the lower is transformed into that of the higher.

Meister Eckhart

To heal is to live one's life as a prayer, accepting our natural state of pure joy and happiness, peace and love, and extending that to all life.

Gerald Tampolsky

Growth Opportunity

Cultivate planned moments for inner silence and meditation. Create moments of silent solitude so your Inner Wisdom can be heard. Learn to be still in the midst of chaos by being alert for spiritually meaningful moments in your active life. Live in a big "now" by being totally present; body, mind, and spirit. Now is the only thing that is real.

The soul is not passive; its energy vibrates in sympathy to us anytime we free ourselves of limitations. A breakthrough of insight stirs the soul, which is felt like a rush of love. There is a similar sense of expansion and liberation when we experience beauty or truth. Always brief, the awakening can change our life. Experiencing a shift in awareness does not have to be a one-time event. As awareness extends it teaches your eyes, your mind and your ego to change. A life committed to deeper awareness becomes a life that creates a new reality. In so doing, we return home to our true Self.

> *Never forget that you are not in the world; the world is in you. Remember who you are. When anything happens to you, take the experience inward. Creation will bring you constant hints and clues about your role as a co-creator. Be aware of them; absorb them. Your soul is metabolizing experience as surely as your body is metabolizing food.*
>
> Deepak Chopra

Application to Nursing Practice

Each of these exercises can be utilized in your life personally, shared with a group of colleagues, or shared with a person or family having a health crisis. Engaging them in a larger conversation will help them discern assumptions and pattern related to their current situation.

Checking In

An essential feature of inner development is the art of being aware of our thoughts and behaviors in the present moment. Learning to "stay awake" allows us to purposefully guide our thinking, emotions and our actions. Then, when we turn off internal dialogue for brief periods of silence, we access our deeper wisdom, intuition, imagination and creativity. Full understanding occurs in silence.

Redirecting your attention:

- Before going to sleep at night, review your day from morning until bedtime.
- Hour by hour, event by event, review the activities and thoughts you experienced.
- At first you may have difficulty remembering.
  - You may be tempted to stop at a specific event and go deeply into it.
  - You may want to criticize an action you took and rewrite the script.
  - You may want to correct some words you said and image an alternative scenario.
  - Resist each temptation and imagine yourself a neutral witness to the events under review.
- In time this exercise will become easier as you develop new powers of alertness and concentration.
- As your evening reflection improves, you will enhance your ability to witness your thoughts and actions as they occur during the day.
- In time you will be able to catch your negative reactions before they manifest.

Cultivating inner silence. A silent mind can be cultivated in many ways:

- Notice your internal conversation. Stop in mid-sentence and go blank. Within a few seconds your internal commentator will speak again, living out another private stage play with friends, enemies or both. When you catch it happening again, go blank again.
- Once you can repeatedly enter that space, even for very brief periods, listen for the silence. At first you may hear subtle vibration caused by your physiology. Simply intend to listen past that sound to find the silence, the quiet place of origin. You may touch it briefly and drift off. Practice will give you a prolonged connection with it, and from that space you will get a direct knowing from your intuition regarding ideas or questions you may have. Trust them.

As you catch and redirect your thoughts in a positive way you redirect your life. And when silence can be experienced true intelligence operates. Stillness is where insight, creativity, and solutions to problems are found.

A Living Story

"Everyone who knows me says I lived a charmed life," says Pauline, a professional woman in her forties. "Some shake their heads and say it enviously, but almost no one knows the truth. There's a reason everything goes right for me. I haven't had a setback in twenty years. Things that look like problems always turn out well in the end. No matter what!

It all goes back to a very stressful time in my life. At age 25 I was out of college with no direction to my life, I had a meaningless secure job and mediocre relationship. Restless and disillusioned, I awoke one night gasping for breath, like someone drowning. Nobody knew what I was feeling or what was going on, and I didn't have anyone to talk to about it. I was breaking up—reshuffling inside. I think the process may have started in childhood actually. I sat by the window in an old armchair, my mind racing. I can't remember what my thoughts were about, but I recall wondering if this is how people lose their minds. The funny thing is that I wasn't agitated emotionally. A strange calm settled over me. I felt like I was watching someone else's mind racing faster and faster.

Suddenly it all stopped. I looked outside at the bright summer sun, and I KNEW "everything you want is coming to you: there is nothing to do." Just like that I felt as if somebody was communicating with me, God, my Higher Self. My body became very relaxed, I thought I was going to cry, but instead, gave an enormous sigh. A huge burden was lifted I didn't even know I was carrying.

After a few days of euphoria I settled down, but I had complete trust in what the voice told me. I had no fear anymore; I saw everything through rose colored glasses. People don't realize it, but fear is always lurking somewhere in the background, like termites in the woodwork. When it's gone the whole world brightens up.

Since that day my life has been beautiful. Bad things stopped happening to me. I started making choices that were right for me. My existence was no longer full of crisis and drama. Other people began to notice that I was living a charmed life." (Chopra 2009, p. 139)

Web Site Resources: What does it mean to really know something as a nursing scientist? To become aware of and consciously include other ways of identifying and considering multiple information sources, you may wish to explore these and other Web sites:

http://www.stevepavlina.com/blog/2006/02/asking-the-right-questions/
http://www.amyscott.com/WAYS%20OF%20KNOWING%20LInking.pdf

BIBLIOGRAPHY

Quotes in the text were taken from the following references:

Berry, C. R. (1988). *When helping you is hurting me: Escaping the Messiah Trap.* Harper & Row.

Campbell, P. (1985). *Bio-spirituality: Focusing as a way to grow.* Chicago, IL: Loyola University Press.

Chopra, D. (2009). *Reinventing the body, resurrecting the soul: How to create a new you.* New York, NY: Harmony Books

Donahue, P. (1989). *Nursing: The finest art.* Boston, MA: Mosby.

Dossey, L. (1982). *Space, time and medicine.* Boston, MA: Shambhala Publications.

Houston, J. (1987). *The search for the beloved.* Houston, TX: Jeremy P. Tarcher.

Klemp, H. (2002). *The spiritual laws of life.* Minneapolis, MN: Eckcankar.

Koerner, J. (2003). *Mother heal myself: An intergenerational healing journey between two worlds.* Santa Rosa, CA: Crestport Press.

Kubler-Ross, E. (1975). *Death: The final stages of growth.* Englewood Cliffs, NJ: Prentice-Hall.

Liberman, J. (1987). *Light: The medicine of the future.* New York, NY: Parabola Books.

Mayeroff, M. (1991). *On caring.* New York, NY: Harper & Row.

Newman, M. (1986). *Health as expanding consciousness.* New York, NY: National League for Nursing.

Palmer, P. (1998). *The courage to teach: Exploring the inner landscape of a teacher's life.* San Francisco, CA: Jossey-Bass Publishers.

Pearson, C. S. (1986). *The hero within: Six archetypes we live by.* New York, NY: Harper & Row.

Peck, S. (1978). *The road less traveled.* Denver, CO: Simon & Schuster.

Prophet, M. L., & Prophet, E. C. (2001). *The masters and the spiritual path.* Corwin Springs, MT: Summit University Press.

Small, J. (1982). *Transformers: The therapists of the future.* Marina del Bay, CA: DeVorss & Company.

Summers, C. (1993). *Inspirations for caregivers.* Mount Shasta, CA: Commune-A-Key Publishing.

Teresa, M. (1996). *Meditations from a simple path*. New York, NY: Ballantine Books.

Tolle, E. (1999). *Practicing the power of now*. Novato, CA: New World Library.

Tolle, E. (2003). *Stillness speaks*. Novato, CA: New World Library.

Tolle, E. (2005). *A new earth: Awakening to your life's purpose*. New York, NY: Penguin Group.

Villoldo, A. (2006). *The four insights: Wisdom, power & grace of the earth-keepers*. Carlsbad, CA: Hay House.

Villoldo, A. (2010). *Illumination: The Shaman's way of healing*. Carlsbad, CA: Hay House.

Woody, C. (2004). *Standing stark: The willingness to engage*. Prescott, AZ: Kenosis Press.

SECTION IV

A HEALING FIELD
THE CONTEXT FOR NURSING PRACTICE

*Happiness is being at peace with your self
while the self is united with a larger
order of things, for we live in the world
which is a sanctuary*

H. Skolimowski

CHAPTER 8

THE NOETIC SCIENTIST
A HOLISTIC WORLDVIEW

Scientists do not invent the truth, they discover it.
Genuine truths exude a beauty,
a rightness, a self-evident quality
that gives them the power of revelation.

John Hogan

Nursing offers us the opportunity to reflect on stories—the stories of others and also the one we are creating as we live our lives fully. Although it is important to identify the major characters and themes that create the scenarios of life, the drama of our lived experience is couched within a larger story—the story of the evolution of the world. It is this silent backdrop, which, while subtle and often unrecognized, forms our understanding of how the world works and our place within it. Meaning is created in this dance between our story and the metastory of scientific evolution—our context for professional practice.

We are living in the twilight of the scientific age. Conventional science is a science of objects; its theories regard objects in terms of other more fundamental objects whose behavior and outcomes can be controlled with predictability. Although the scientific community differs on their answers to the question, "what is life beyond biological functioning?" scientific advances pose increasing limitations upon itself. Ironically, as scientific discovery progresses it is beginning to realize the ultimate *limits of knowledge*; science, as Hogan (1996) has put it, may be ending because it has worked so well.

Increasingly, scientists from various disciplines cast their gaze across the field and find that, for all its power and richness, it cannot explain the ultimate mystery of consciousness; the link between mind and matter. The enlarging voice of quantum physicists postulates that the key to this deep divide lies in the fissure between two major theories of modern physics: quantum mechanics (which describes nuclear forces) and electromagnetism and general relativity; Einstein's theory of gravity (Penrose, 1994).

EXPANDING OUR SCIENCE: HOLISM VERSUS REDUCTIONISM

For the past 400 years, Western Civilization has looked to science as its source of truth and wisdom regarding the mysteries of life. In 1543, Copernicus' observations regarding reality began a scientific revolution that was later defined by Newton. The Newtonian classical physic-based deterministic worldview fostered a materialistic mindset that saw the world as an intricate mechanism with separate parts and processes. The scientist's job was to discover the thread that unifies and weaves the separate entities into a unified whole through a process of *reductionism*—taking matter apart and studying its bits and pieces. In this model, *causation flows upward as "matter before mind"* from the base level of elementary particles (Goswami, 2004).

Elementary particles create atoms, which in turn form molecules that configure together to produce a cell. Cells generate all of the energies of the body. Some of the cells create neurons which in turn construct the brain. The brain generates mental processes in the upper levels of hierarchy. Knowledge of the universe's parts and their interaction allows scientists to predict and control nature. Control is the principle function of *determinism*, the belief that with knowledge of something's parts we can predict its behavior. This materialistic and deterministic worldview fosters a dualistic perspective; a split between mind and matter which can be controlled and managed through the "laws of science." It supports the idea that humans are disconnected from, and above, nature.

This reductionistic approach to understanding the nature of the universe has bestowed the valuable knowledge that created the space age and artificial hearts and limbs and deciphered the genetic code. However, applying those same principles to business, health care, and world problems is hastening our demise. Therefore, leading-edge scientific research is beginning to question fundamental assumptions long held as dogma by conventional science.

The discovery of the quantum world put an end to certainty. Prigogine and other scientists noted that chaos and complexity offer a different vision of the world from the mechanistic view of traditional science. This world is filled with fluidity, multiplicity, plurality, connectedness, segmentarity, heterogeneity, and resilience. *Downward causation of "mind over matter"* originates from the intentions and thoughts of the individual rather than some outside force. The notion of "scientific knowledge" is replaced with the concept of '*self-organizing dynamics*' of nonorganic, organic, and social phenomena. Determinism is replaced with *emergence* of new order as this chaotic phenomenon is supported, rather than controlled, by links between order and disorder as new form materializes (Prigogine & Stengers, 1984). The underlying assumption is that to understand nature and the human experience we must transcend the parts to see the interconnected whole.

The impact of a radically new worldview challenges the very foundations of medical and nursing practice. Western medicine traditionally conceptualized the body as a grand machine, controlled by the brain and peripheral nervous system; the ultimate biological computer. Human physiology and psychological behavior were viewed as dependent on the structure and hardware of brain and body, with a mechanical heart pump to deliver nutrients to all body cells.

This traditional viewpoint is expanding since Einstein's discovery introduced the concept that all matter is an expression of energy. Einstein stepped beyond reductionism towards holism, showing that both matter and energy are expressions of the same universal substance (Einstein, 1952). The recognition that all matter is energy, $E = mc^2$, forms the foundation for understanding how human beings can be considered dynamic energetic systems. In this world, human beings are viewed as networks of complex energy fields that interface with physical/cellular systems (McTaggart, 2002). Therefore, healing of this basic vibrational energetic level of substance can be accomplished through multiple therapeutic venues such as therapeutic touch, homeopathy, and acupuncture.

In spite of a growing field of evidence, present day Newtonian models of medical thinking still prevail in the practice of conventional medicine, the context for contemporary nursing practice. We are being called to re-vision our world and our work by embracing the best of tradition while expanding our worldview to encompass the larger quantum world of holism.

ENLARGING OUR PRACTICE—EXPANSIVE SCIENTIFIC MODELS

Lipton (2005–2006) notes that over the centuries scientists have constructed their knowledge into a hierarchical, multitiered building. Each level, distinguished by a specific subspecialty, is built upon the supporting structures of lower levels. We are now invited to "enlarge our 'living room'" by incorporating the tools and processes of the quantum world into our world and our work.

The *foundation for integrative science is laid on the first floor of fractals and chaos.* Mathematical laws have traditionally been used to isolate and divide the universe into separate measurable components. Future science will also include the emerging new math that emphasizes the disciplines of fractal geometry, chaos theory and fuzzy logic (Kosko, 1993). Bohm also suggests that the new research tool is dialogue rather than statistics. In true dialogue, multiple perspectives are shared and something organic, "emerging, and new" is discovered in the shared space (Bohm & Peat, 1987).

Fractals, the modern version of geometry, were defined by IBM scientist Benoit Mandelbrot (1977). This simple mathematic equation involves addition and multiplication, with the results being entered back into the original equation and solved again. Repetition of the equation provides for a geometric expression of self-similar objects that appear at higher or lower levels of magnitude. Like nested Russian dolls, organization at any level of nature reflects a self-similar pattern at higher and lower levels of reality. The structure and function of a cell reflects behavior of a human, group and society. "As above, so below" is emphasized, showing that the observable physical universe is derived from the interconnectivity and integration of all its parts.

Displacing the Darwinian evolution theory based on mutations and a struggle for survival, fractal geometry demonstrates that the biosphere is a very structured and cooperative venture amongst all living organisms. Rather than competition for survival, nature models cooperation amongst species living in harmony with their environment. It highlights the fact that every being counts; we are all members of a single organism.

The dynamics of fractal structures, from mountains to clouds to plants to humans, are directly influenced by chaos theory (Gribbon, 2004). This math transcends predictability and control, showing that a small change may cause unexpected final outcomes. Combining chaos theory with fractal geometry, the behavioral dynamics in physical reality can only be predicted within a reference range of possible outcomes rather than controlled.

The *second floor of science explores energy physics*. A century ago a group of creative minorities in the field of quantum mechanics transcended the Newtonian view of the universe as an assembly of physical parts. Albert Einstein, Max Planck and Werner Heisenberg, among others, revealed that there is no true "physicality" in the universe (Hawking, 1988). Atoms are miniature tornados of energy, popping in and out of existence. They create energy fields that encompass the universe, closely entangled with each other and the field that contains them all.

A radical conclusion of the new physics recognizes that "the observer influences the observed object by the act of observing it." Observations are influenced by the sensibilities which inform our perception; the universe is a "mental" construct.

Physicist Sir James Jean observed that "The stream of knowledge is heading toward a nonmechanical reality; the universe begins to look more like a great thought than like a great machine." (Henry, 2005) While this knowledge was uncovered 80 years ago, many scientists cling rigidly to the prevailing matter-oriented worldview. We are being called to recognize that our beliefs, perceptions, and attitudes about the world create that world for us.

The *third floor of science focuses on vibrational chemistry*. Conventional chemistry was built on atomic elements of solid electrons, protons and neutrons within a Newtonian solar system. Vibrational chemistry is derived from quantum mechanics which view atoms as spinning immaterial energy vortices called quarks. It sees vibration as the process which creates molecular bonds and drives molecular interactions. Energy fields, such as those emerging from outside sources like cell phones, or the interior world of thoughts and emotions, interact with and influence chemical reactions (Rasha, 2003).

Mind–body connection is mediated by the mechanisms fostered by vibrational chemistry. The body is created from a hundred thousand different protein molecules which change shape in response to signals. These harmonic vibrations in the field influence the collective movement of the protein body, generating the behaviors we observe as "life."

Life controlling signals originate from physical chemicals as well as energy waves. This energy–protein interface is the junction of the mind–body connection. (Pert, 1997)

The *fourth floor of science focuses on the new biology*. In traditional biology, in reductionistic fashion, organisms are dissected into cells and molecular parts to gain understanding of how they work. The new science perceives cells as integrated communities that are physically and energetically entangled within their environment (Gerber, 1996). James Lovelock's hypothesis states that our Earth and its biosphere comprise a single living and breathing entity, Gaia. Gaian philosophy emphasizes participation and integration of all the earth's organisms to maintain homeostasis and balance (Lovelock, 1979).

A second new field on biology is the power of epigenetics. This field, which means "control above the genes," addresses the newly uncovered second genetic code that controls the activity and programming of DNA. A heredity mechanism, it reveals how behavior and gene activity are controlled by the organism's perception of its environment. Moving from the determinism of DNA coding, epigenetics recognizes the role of our perceptions, including emotions and consciousness, in controlling our genes. Applied consciousness can be used to shape our biology, making us "masters" of our own lives (Lipton, 2005).

The *fifth floor of science focuses on energy psychology*. For centuries our materialistic perspective has dismissed the immaterial mind and consciousness, perceiving instead that our genes and neurochemicals—the hardware of our central nervous system—were responsible for behavior and dysfunction alike. Quantum mechanics, vibrational chemistry, and epigenetics offer a new understanding of psychology.

The environment, coupled with perceptions of the mind and their resultant emotions and feelings, control behavior and genetics. Our lives are controlled by our perceptions of life experiences rather than by genetic programming (Mindel, 2004). Moving from Newtonian to quantum mechanics shifts the focus of psychology from physiochemical mechanisms to energy fields. This altered understanding moves us from psychological interventions targeted at physiochemical hardware, genetic manipulation, or altered physiology and behavior modification.

An enlarged focus on energy psychology recognizes the power of fundamental perceptions, leading to the creation of deepening developmental experiences as a therapeutic intervention. An encounter that offers new perspective enhances our health, intelligence and happiness, shifting our values and moral code to a higher order. Focusing on our potential and our capacity moves us forward into a fuller life, rather than backwards to a limiting history.

By remodeling each "floor" of our house of science, we strengthen the building while adding an observatory on the top. From this vantage point our worldview is holistic; the view of a *noetic scientist*. The word "noetic," coming from ancient Greece, refers to an "inner knowing," an intuitive consciousness which is direct and immediate; accessing us to knowledge beyond what is available to our normal senses and our patterns of reasoning, (www.noetic.org). Here we "know" that the physical character of atoms, proteins, cells and people are all influenced by immaterial energies that form a collective field. Each human, a collective cellular community, responds to a unique spectrum of the universe's energy field. This unique spectrum, referred to by many as Spirit, signifies an invisible moving force that is in harmonic resonance with our physical body. This profound, creative force behind consciousness shapes our physical reality.

We also note that collectively we are a part of a larger, shared field that cocreates our reality. As this understanding deepens, our relationship with the planet becomes one of partnership. We begin to live lightly on the earth, using only the resources we need while practicing principles that support sustainability. We live responsibly, moving with care and compassion through the world.

RECREATING OUR REALITY—NURSES AS NOETIC SCIENTISTS

To resolve local and global crisis requires us to re-vision conventional science through the integration and coordination of both the physical/material world and the energetic/immaterial world. Deep healing and wholeness will come through the support and services of *cultural creatives*, a minority of healers who practice from an integrative view of themselves and the world.

We live in a time of great promise as we have developed economic and social systems that tap human creativity as never before. The dilemma of our time is the fact that we lack the broader social and economic systems to fully harness human creativity and put it to best use.

The number of people doing creative work that will transform society has been steadily increasing, especially in the past two decades. These pioneers of the new age, working as scientists, engineers, artists, and knowledge-based professionals such as nurses, are referred to as the "Creative Class."

Creative nurses have always been in our midst, living an experiential lifestyle. Our history is rich with their presence, starting with Florence Nightingale. The foundation for nursing's work is first and foremost science; applied science is our practice domain. The mindset of a contemporary scientist is reflected in the clinical reasoning capacity of this nurse. The nurse is focused on finding answers that produce an outcome: she or he cannot tolerate untestable speculation. The creative is eager to share their knowledge in an effort to make things as clear as possible, and to test and expand understanding by networking with similar colleagues. Free of self-doubt, wishful thinking, and deep attachment to specific theories or protocols, this applied scientist simply comes from a stance of wanting to know how things work to create a positive affect for the patient.

A study by Rich Florida (2002) demonstrated that in 1900 less than 1% of American workers were doing creative work. By 1980 the figure was still well below 10%. Today, more than 30% of the nation's workforce is shaping the profound transformation in the ways we work, in our values and desires, and the very fabric of our lives. Capacities of those who "live on the edge" as agents of change inside traditional professional jobs include

- *Technology*: These nurses embrace, seek out and create solutions that utilize emerging smart technologies (new tools and resources—both material and ideological) to extend their capacity. Rather than nursing the technology, they use the technology's information and power to serve both the patient and themselves.
- *Talent*: These nurses not only demonstrate clinical and technical skill and aptitude, but a creative and adventuresome capacity for innovation and experimentation.

- *Tolerance*: These nurses have an edge in the ability to attract different kinds of people who generate new ideas and methods for responding to the work before them. They thrive on diversity and change, using the chaos and energy to further their own experimentation and contribution to the larger field.

Cultural creatives engage an active imagination. Quantum scientist Minsky confessed he would love to know what Yo-Yo Ma felt as he was playing a concert, doubting whether such an experience were possible. To do so he would have to have all of Yo-Yo Ma's memories, he would have to *become* Yo-Yo Ma. But in becoming Yo-Yo Ma, he would cease to be Minsky. No such reduction is possible because multiplicity of the mind is the human birthright.

The cultural creatives, having mastered many skills during their career, enjoy "the feeling of awkwardness" triggered by having to learn something new. There is no sense of failure when things do not work out, rather the delight of experimentation and discovery that is present in children. Minsky further stated, "It's so thrilling not to be able to do something. It's such a rare experience to treasure, and it won't last long" (Hogan, 1996, pp. 188–189). He observed that the most important thing in life is to grow beyond our current state, to become more our essential authentic self. This is the grand opportunity called "life."

Resourceful nurses thrive in a broad ecosystem that nourishes and supports creativity and channels it into innovation that eventually changes practice within the discipline.

Such nurses have always worked on the margins, expanding the field on behalf of the people we are privileged to serve. The key to their survival is to "squelch the squelchers"; the controlling leaders, micromanagers, and broader structures of social control and vertical power. The real threat to America is not terrorism, but rather the suppression of the creative and talented people who have a commitment and capacity to enrich the world in which we live.

The power of this cultural scientific revolution lies in a nurse's ability to select the "best-of-breed" ideas and innovations and blend them in novel ways. People with differing perspectives contribute their own original ideas into the boiling stew, creating new thought. Connection and collaboration are the tools of the information age that are essential for the creatives in our midst.

Just as cultural advancement learned to operate independently of biological evolution, so too is web-based progression becoming autonomous. For thousands of years human progress was limited to the very slow pace of genetic evolution. Cultural scientific evolution is much faster because what is learned can be passed on through language. Beginning with the development of the alphabet and then the printing press, the emergence of the internet has put wings on communication in ways that transcend time and distance.

The intellectual impact of this interconnected world is fostering a Renaissance greater than any shift in the history of humankind. Even scientists and specialists are increasingly taking the real-time word of electronic circuits for critical information on vital issues.

By processing information adaptively, the nurse of the twenty-first century will open up important new vistas for health and healing to the people she or he serves. Patients and families will absorb new, enhanced information through their health care experience, adjusting themselves accordingly. Their tomorrows will turn out differently from their today's, for increased understanding leaves us free to evolve in whatever fashion works best for each of us. And in the process of shared growth and understanding, the world will become a healing place.

I will not die an unlived life.
I will not live in fear
Of falling or catching fire.
I choose to inhabit my days,
To allow my living to open me,
To make me less afraid,
More accessible,
To loosen my heart
Until it becomes a wing,
A torch, a promise.
I choose to risk my significance;
To live so that which came to me as seed
Goes to the next as blossom
And that which came to me as blossom,
Goes on as fruit.

Dawna Markova

Applying the Concepts in Nursing

The scientific process is a cornerstone of nursing practice. We are expert at its application through use of the Nursing Process. A Noetic Nurse Scientist realizes that the most expansive solution begins with the right question. What you are looking for/at determines what your outcome will be. You are invited to pay careful attention to the question that you are asking; you can increase your problem-solving skills at work and at home by honing your question-asking ability.

Checking In

Review your history of questioning/decision making: Where and when have you made clear-cut decisions? What was the result? If things didn't turn out the way I had planned, what did I learn? How did the experience enrich my life? Where and when have I simply stated preferences and hoped they would come about without making clear commitment? What was the result? How can I shift my thinking to make clear-cut, definite, and effective decisions? When I have made a clear-cut decision, how have I followed through with that decision? Do I need to make adjustments in my follow-up?

You can you sharpen your question-asking/decision-making skills so that new and deeper solutions can come to you. Begin by asking the simple, 'naïve' questions that sophisticated minds often overlook. Why is this a problem? Is this the real issue? Why have we always done it this way? Your aim is to raise questions that have not been asked before prior to selecting a solution.

Begin by "identifying" the problem. What is the problem? Are there underlying issues? What preconceptions, prejudices, or paradigms may be influencing my perceptions? What will happen if I ignore the problem? What possibilities may exist that I haven't yet considered? What problems may be caused by solving this problem? What metaphors from nature can I use to illuminate it?

A PROBLEM-SOLVING CHECKLIST

- WHEN did it start? Does it happen? Doesn't it happen? Will the consequences of it be felt? Must it be resolved?

- WHO cares about it? Is affected by it? Created it? Perpetuates it? Can help solve it?
- HOW does it happen? Can I get more objective information? Can I look at it from unfamiliar perspectives? Can it be changed? Will I know that It has been solved?
- WHERE does it happen? Did it begin? Haven't I looked? Else has the happen?
- WHY is it important? Did it start? Does it continue? Ask why, why, why, why, why.....to get to the bottom of an issue.

> *Leonardo da Vinci was not content to record how a thing worked: he wished to find out why. It is this curiosity which transformed a technician into a scientist.*
>
> K. Clark

A Living Example

The history of the world is filled with examples of the evolution of ideas and societies by individuals and groups that have expanding what is possible for their society. Questions can be framed in a wide variety of ways, and the 'framing' dramatically influences the ability to find appropriate solutions.

Nomadic society moved within a geographic region based on their needs for survival, looking for food, shelter, and water. Their lives were prompted by the question "How do we get to water?" Well-known paths to the water sources in their area helped them provide this essential resource to the tribe. They lived and moved amongst these various sites as seasons and conditions allowed.

Suddenly, an evolution in their questioning resulted in a major transformation of human society. Instead of following the predictable and known, someone restated the question: "How do we get the water to come to us?" Reframing the question began the development of community infrastructures that moved society towards stability and the evolution of an agrarian society.

Web site Resources: To explore your critical analysis abilities and gain a richer perspective and deeper understanding of concepts and issues regarding asking the right questions, refer to these Web sites: *http://www.stevepavlina.com/blog/2006/02/asking-the-right-questions/ http://catb.org/~esr/faqs/smart-questions.html*

BIBLIOGRAPHY

Bohm, D., & Peat, E. F. (1987). *Science, order and creativity.* New York, NY: Bantam Books.

Einstein, A. (1952). *The principle of relativity: A collection of original papers on the special and general theory of relativity.* New York, NY: Dover.

Florida, R. (2002). *The rise of the creative class: And how it's transforming work, leisure, community & everyday life.* New York, NY: Basic Books.

Gerber, R. (1996). *Vibrational medicine.* Santa Fe, NM: Bear & Company.

Goswami, A. (2004). *The quantum doctor: A physicist's guide to health and healing.* Charlottesville, VA: Hampton Roads Publishing Company.

Gribbin, J. (2004). *Deep simplicity: Chaos, complexity and the emergence of life* (p. 215). London, UK: Allan Lane.

Hawking, S. (1988). *A brief history of time: From the big bang to black holes.* London, UK: Bantam Press.

Henry, R. C. (2005). The mental universe, *Nature, 436,* 29.

Hogan, J. (1996). *The end of science.* New York, NY: Broadway Books.

Kosko, B. (1993). *Fuzzy thinking: The new science of fuzzy logic.* New York, NY: Hyperion.

Lipton, B. (2005). *The biology of belief: Unleashing the power of consciousness, matter and miracles.* Santa Rosa, CA: Mountain of Love/Elite Books.

Lipton, B. (2005–2006). Embracing the immaterial universe. *Shift: At the Frontiers of Consciousness,* 4(9), 8–12.

Lovelock, J. (1979). *Gaia: A new look at life on earth.* Oxford, UK: Oxford University Press.

Mandelbrot, B. (1977). *The fractal geometry of nature.* San Francisco, CA: W. H. Freeman.

McTaggart, L. (2002). *The field.* New York, NY: HarperCollins Publisher.

Mindel, A. (2004). *The quantum mind and healing.* Charlottesville, VA: Hampton Roads Publishing Company.

Penrose, R. (1994). *Shadows of the mind.* New York, NY: Oxford University Press.

Pert, C. (1997). *Molecules of emotion: Why you feel the way you feel.* New York, NY: Scribner.

Prigogine, I., & Stengers, I. (1984). *Order out of chaos.* New York, NY: Bantam Books.

Rasha, (2003). *Oneness.* Santa Fe, NM: Earthstar Press.

CHAPTER 9

THE CREATIVE ARTIST
COMPOSING A LIFE

Einstein's space is no closer to reality than Van Gogh's sky. The glory of science is not in a truth more absolute than the truth of Bach or Tolstoy, but in the act of creation itself. The scientist's discoveries impose his own order on chaos, as the composer or painter imposes his; an order that always refers to limited aspects of reality, and is based on the observer's frame of reference, which differs from period to period as a Rembrandt nude differs from a nude by Manet.

Arthur Koestler

Nightingale identified nursing as the "finest of arts" often in her powerful reflections on the discipline. Cocreating a life-altering experience with the person facing a health crisis has been the hallmark of our trade. What comprises that subtle, but profound, aspect of professional practice that includes but transcends the scientific rigor we bring to the patient encounter? We are practicing the trade secrets of an artist, a person whose creative work shows sensitivity and imagination.

Each of us is born into a culture whose orientations and basic convictions shape us, remaining deeply rooted in our subconscious for all of our life. We carry the messages and rules of family, friends, and authority figures deep in our belief system, cheering or scolding from the balcony of our mind as we navigate the world. As we move beyond home and hearth, we find differing cultures and beliefs that we can incorporate into our understanding of the world. However, those first roots remain deep and immovable, no matter how we try to shake or transcend them.

This same phenomenon is observed within a field of knowledge. Various educational endeavors and "first job experiences" burn expectations and attitudes deeply into our personality. Similarly, the sources that gave birth to a field such as nursing, remain within the profession as a skeleton that organizes the shape of things, defining in part what is real and true, what embodies the basic essence of reality from that point of view.

When we, or a field, encounter new data that contradicts our old beliefs and basic orientation, a struggle of confusion arises. There is increasing difficulty in communication between those within the family or the field. Early adaptors will incorporate some of the new into their world and work, while a small segment will die without ever acknowledging that anything could ever change. For the majority, however, there is a dance between old and new, past and future, with a slow drift toward the pole that attracts us most.

The reality that comprises our world of observation can be divided into differing realms of experience, each with a different level of awareness.

1. *Consensus Reality* is comprised of observations of time, space, and matter experienced through repeatable shared experiences and behaviors. Cause-and-effect activities of things that can be seen or touched comprise this domain, which is validated by the science and culture of the times. We engage with this *outer world,* reacting or responding based on decisions made as "The Evaluator."

2. *Inner Reality* is comprised of highly individualized analysis of outer world experiences through intuition, subjective feelings, emotions, and dreams. We create meaning from *inner world* projections and interpretations that we selectively or habitually weave into our experiences in patterned fashion. Depicted through the contributions of the arts, we experience this world as "The Interpreter."

3. *Core Essence* is a perception of the subtle energy field behind the form being observed. In this space is a clear sense of the qualities that comprise the thing, that is, the "essence of flowers" with color, shape, and size varying while all hold a fragrance, a fragile beauty and vulnerability; the "essence of cat" with size, color, and pedigree varying while all hold an attitude of

owning their master. An unspoken recognition of "qualities" emerges from a flash of insight as the mysterious reveals itself in the silence from which all things arise; including an awareness of things too big to be touched (macrocosm), as well as those too small to be seen (microcosm). This field is the Universal sacred space of Spirit addressed by philosophy and religion. To perceive this world requires us to become "The Witness" to things invisible that cannot be named.

Science explores the reality of the physical world while art focuses on experiences of inner reality. Philosophy and religion give shape and direction to the realm of essence, influencing the moral ethics of the times (Leshan & Margenau, 1982). Together, these things form and inform, bringing beauty and meaning to the human journey. Each of these realms is experienced uniquely as an individual, and collectively as the human family. But the ongoing explorations and discoveries in art, science and philosophy keep redefining these domains, inviting us to continue expanding our own capacities for understanding, creating an expansion of consciousness.

Art and physics fashion a strange partnership, yet they are the forces that define and unite our objective and subjective worlds together. The artist creates a world of image and metaphor while the physicist employs numbers and equations. Art embraces the imaginative reality of aesthetic qualities while physics shuttles between a world of specific mathematical relationships and quantifiable properties. Art creates illusions to elicit emotion while physics strives to create an exact and predictable science. However, when closely examined, both are an effort at investigating the nature of reality to create an understanding of "life" more fully. Noted physicist David Bohm observed that "Physics is a form of insight and as such it's a form of art" (Shlain, 1991, p. 78).

Although the scientific side of nursing practice breaks things into component parts to establish a relationship between them, the artist intuitively arranges distinct and unique features and patterns of the particular patient and his or her circumstance into a larger whole. The witness discerns timing and tempo, creating a rhythm in the process that keeps tempo with the song of the soul. There is considerable creative crossover in this sacred work of addressing the wholeness of the situation and all involved (Anodea, 2004).

ART—THE POWER OF PERSPECTIVE

Radical innovations in art embody the preverbal stages of new concepts that hold potential to change the outcome of an external event, group or society. A new way to think about reality begins with the recognition or assimilation of unfamiliar images. These new thoughts and possibilities lead to abstract ideas that later give rise to specific words and/or actions. When we reflect, reminisce, ruminate and imagine we are generally in the visual mode. However, to perform the brain's highest function, abstract thought, we must move to the realm of essence; energy before form. Here we go beyond the use of images, engaging our intuition and intent to create in a world that transcends image and language.

Notably, it is images that precede abstract thought and descriptive language. Artist Paul Klee observed that "The artist does not reproduce the visible; rather he makes things visible" (Chipp, 1956, p. 182). Picasso said, "I see for others" (Reed, 1968, p. 87). Nurses are both artist in their trade, and observer in the gallery of another's masterpiece—their life. When they enter the nurse–patient experience with respect for the person, the nurse recognizes that, as their own life artist the person has crafted their journey in the way that seems best to them. Without judgment, the compassionate professional stands alongside the person and family as they view the situation at hand, incorporating new information and issues into the landscape of their existence. Goethe observed (Dowson, 1979, p. 26):

> Works of art specify no immediate action or limited use. They are like gateways, where the visitor [nurse as witness] can enter the space of the artist [patient-family], or the time of the poet [context-culture], to experience whatever rich domain [life] the artist has fashioned.

Art and physics, like wave and particle, weave together to form an articulation of the clinical reasoning process which gives the "interpreter" function of nursing a profound place of importance in the healing experience. This recognition of an understated phenomenon and an immediate proactive response can alter the ultimate outcome and future state for all involved (Pesut & Herman, 1999).

Multidimensionality—The Influence of Time and Space

One of the great gifts of art is the opportunity to see the world through perspectives other than our own. Many artistic styles have evolved throughout history, depicting our deepening perception of time and space, and humankinds place within it. Their enlarging view influences our own, much like a healing presence potentiates new possibility for the patient and family.

A *zero-dimensional world* is expressed in the simplest geometric object; a point. Without size, it can only be imagined. It fixes a location in space with a dimension that equals zero. When this point gets extended into a simple line, it has only *one dimension*—length. One-dimensional perception views the world as connected points only, with nothing residing outside those points.

A *two-dimensional world* includes the concept of a plane— a surface. In this universe things have breadth and width, while still lacking height. Some of the early art forms created on the walls of cave dwellings were depicted in the form of stick figures and objects. A two-dimensional world encounters lines, or barriers, with time experienced as the "moment." Since this space is a flatland, any barrier must be walked around, for there is no "space" to jump or step over the object.

Third-dimensional space includes matter—a solid body that adds the perspective of height or mass, and linear time marching progressively forward. The generation of Renaissance painters perfected the depiction of a broad view from a single perspective by incorporating the third dimension in depth painting. In these art forms an object painted on a flat surface was given the perception of depth by making objects appear to have the same size, shape and position in relation to each other. In such a picture the road diminishes in size and prominence as it moves back into the horizon, while smaller trees dot the background with the larger in the foreground. Great masters, including such notables as Da Vinci and Michelangelo, left many images of beauty for us in this three-dimensional realm of length, breadth and depth (Shlain, 1991, p. 24) (Figure 9.1).

A three-dimensional being can see only two dimensions while humans can note all three. Because we can delineate external forms in three dimensions and manipulate three-dimensional

FIGURE 9.1

Dimensions of Space Time

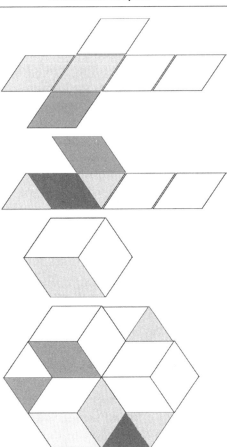

spaces, we must recognize the truth; that we are *four-dimensional beings* (Steiner, 2001, pp. 8–10, 40–42).

By adding the fourth dimension of multiple possibilities, everyday three-dimensional space is transformed into a four-dimensional hyperspace that is infused with an unlimited vista including the past, the future and the timeless. In this extending view, you become aware of your "observer self" witnessing a larger reality. You begin to note an ongoing process moving between and through yourself as well as all other states of being.

A recent Norman Rockwell art exhibit featured some of his most famous works. Instead of the traditional art show of original paintings, this exhibit also offered several life-size models built to allow the viewer to enter the picture, interact with it and experience it from multiple perspectives.

The story captured in the picture, *Surprise,* which appeared on the Saturday Evening Post cover in March, 1956, occurs in a one-room schoolhouse. You enter the school through the back door, stepping behind several rows of desks to the backs of the children facing a blackboard. Miss Jones is standing in front of the room, gazing at the children with delight and affection mirrored in her eyes. The blackboard holds multiple messages of "Surprise" and "Happy Birthday Miss Jones," "Miss Jones is our favorite teacher," and so on.

Walking down the aisle, you may stop and sit in a student desk. When the desk lid is lifted, one sees a small slate blackboard, chalk, books and a wide-awake toad that was captured at recess. Arriving at the front of the room, you may take your place beside Miss Jones and see the excitement and joy on the faces of the children. Opening her desk you find a collection of teaching materials, along with an abundance of slingshots and paper wads with rubber bands. You may write on the board, adding your own greeting to this beloved teacher.

After you have walked through and experienced the perspective of each of the major characters in the picture, you have a deep and rich sense of what it must have been like to be both the student and teacher in an era of greater simplicity. You may recall similar moments in your own childhood, whether at school or with grand/parents, when you crafted a surprise to show appreciation for someone's guiding presence in your life. An artifact in a desk or on the wall can trigger emotions and thoughts that have not been examined for many years. You may recall your own school experiences, or ponder how vastly different the education of your grandchildren will be with the advent of the Internet and the ease of global travel.

As you walk through the painting, you select items of interest. You and each object you relate to are intimate, connected in a pure and intimate way. You become both yourself and the object toward which you move. In the end, you have reflected on something larger than yourself, a phenomenon that spans both time and distance. Deeper understanding and meaning are possible from this point of view (Malcolm, 1994, p. 31).

In *fourth-dimensional space,* half of the experience—objects and the light that illumines them—are objectively given. The other two dimensions, emotions and interpretation, are subjectively experienced. The further we move into other dimensions, the more subjective the experience becomes. What lies within the higher worlds can only be attained through the development of new "envisioning possibilities." We must become active in accessing and understanding these worlds, rather than passive viewers only.

Physicists are now exploring "hyperspace" and have identified as many as 10 differing dimensions, including wormholes, superstrings and parallel universes (Kaku, 1994). Although mathematicians, physicists, and computers have no problem solving theoretical problems in multidimensional space, humans find it impossible to visualize universes beyond their own four-dimensional world.

Artist photographers are giving us new images of the macrocosm with pictures from the Hubble spacecraft that are startling in their beauty and magnitude. Contemporary film-makers working with computer-assisted graphics are creating compelling epic movies, such as *Lord of the Rings,* and *Harry Potter,* endowing humans with super-human capacities. Popular motion pictures also create awareness of things unseen through stories, such as *Avatar* and *The Matrix.* Action-oriented art forms such as these are heralding a new way of being in multiple worlds simultaneously, opening up and modeling new possibilities and capacities for the next generation of humanity.

One fundamental theme running through the findings in physics over the past decade is this: "The laws of nature become simpler and more elegant when expressed in higher dimensions, which is their natural home" (Kaku, 1994 p. 12). In higher order, as the number of dimensions in space time increase, more forces can be accommodated. Here we have enough "room" to unify all of the known physical forces; electromagnetic, strong nuclear, weak nuclear, and gravitational forces. When these laws, which seem to have no relationship in three-dimensional space, are viewed in their natural habitat in the dimensions beyond space and time, their true brilliance and power can be observed and appreciated. The laws become simple and powerful and beautiful. Beauty is the hallmark of Truth.

The revolution sweeping over physics is the realization that we do not have the technology or the money to "prove" (in the traditional sense) the reality of these far-reaching dimensions. Because it is untestable, scientists are asking this question: "*Is beauty, by itself, a physical principle that can be substituted for the lack of experimental verification?*" (Kaku, 1994, p. 179). Suddenly, the physicist is an artist!

Western Science is a young 400 years old, while art is ancient, preceding the emergence of language amongst the human species. And both are moving back/forward to a "natural" connection with the nature of all life. Abram has observed that "without the oxygenating breath of the forests, the clutch of gravity, we have no distance from our technologies, no way of assessing their limitations, no way of keeping ourselves from turning into them....only when we are in regular contact with the tangible ground and sky can we learn how to orient and to navigate in the multiple dimensions that now claim us." (Abram, 1996, p. x) This is the gift of the artist; they give life and articulation to the essence of things of nature and spirit.

PATTERN—THE POWER OF LIMITS

The nurse artist has an exceptional capacity to recognize pattern and rhythm, as well as typical modifications induced by illness. She has taken an innate gift possessed by all at birth and enhanced a capacity for its application in professional practice.

Apple blossoms always have five petals and hands host five digits. When we look deeply into the patterns of a blossom, a seashell, or a song we discover a perfection of order that reveals an infinity greater than our own. Between the borders of art, science, religion, and philosophy lies a power that shapes our universe, our lives and our values: the golden mean. "The proportions in art, nature, and the human body are shared limitations that create harmonious relationships out of differences. Limitations are not just restrictive, they are also creative" (Doczi, 1994) (Figure 9.2).

There is discipline inherent in the patterns of natural phenomena, manifest in the most ageless and harmonious works of man in art, music, architecture, and social systems. Order emerges as certain proportions appear again and again, showing a dynamic growth pattern through a union of complementary opposites. Old

FIGURE 9.2

The Golden Mean

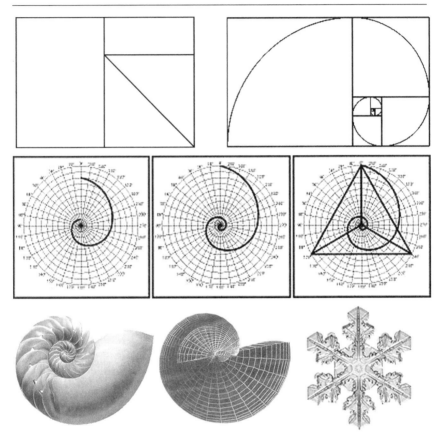

and new stages of growth always share the same angles and proportions. The formula of the celebrated *golden mean* A : B = B : (A + B), implies a reciprocal relationship between two unequal parts of a whole, where the smaller part stands in the same proportion to the larger part as the large part stands to the whole (Doczi, 1994, p. 2).

Patterns typically generate spirals that move in opposite directions forming a union of complementary opposites—sun and moon, Yin and Yang, male and female, positive and negative energy. This pattern-forming process creates an energy, a generative power called *dinergy*—the creative energy of organic growth.

This energy-creating process transforms discrepancies into harmonies by allowing differences to complement each other through the power of certain proportions, analogous to musical root harmonies. Its power lies in the unique capacity to unite the differing parts into a whole that preserves the identity of each while blending them into a greater pattern of a single larger whole—an infinite number of times. Herein lays the foundation of cosmic order expressed in numerous mathematical equations and spiritual geometry (Doczi, 1994, p. 13).

Reality unites and diversifies at the same time. Poetry, painting, and the arts are given as a way for us to uncover the unity present in the variety of our human experiences. While there is no event or shape exactly the same, there is none so entirely different from another. Nature accomplishes the most impossible feat: simultaneously creating forms that are both similar and dissimilar, united and diverse. This is what helps us distinguish human from animal and person from person; all are variations of the golden mean's proportions. Its simple aesthetic contribution is based on its direct relation to order and its inverse relation to complexity (Doczi, 1994, p. 25).

The ratio of dinergy is present in the crafts, the masterfully woven ceremonial blankets of First Nations artists, the delicate painting on a Chinese vase, the proportions of the human body in the sculpture of David. It is heard in musical creations based on a seven tone scale, combined in endless iterations for song and dance and the written word based on shared meaning. The number seven is the primary harmonic quality. There are seven colors in the spectrum of a prism, seven notes in the musical scale, 7 days in the week, seven chakras in the human body. The Lakota Sioux speaks of the seven sacred directions; north, south, east, west, above, below, and the seventh sacred direction of the heart directly connected to Creator.

The ratio of dinergy is present in mathematical calculations from the Fibonacci numbers series to the architectural wonders of the world built from carefully calculated drawings. It is present everywhere in nature, from the pattern in a flower to the design of our DNA. Unity within the diversities of organic and inorganic matter can be seen in the spiral patterns of the galaxies, the tiny spiral pattern found in shells, flowers and pinecones, and the spiral pattern on our fingertips.

The science of nursing is focused on the functioning of the physical body, which is assessed and managed by diagnostic measurements and protocol-driven treatments. The art of nursing is concerned with the subtle aspects of care, noting a shift in pattern, a change in affect, an unstated concern expressed in body movements and facial expression displayed on both the foreground and background of the human landscape.

Leonardo Da Vinci created his famous drawing when the Renaissance rediscovered the classic remains of Greece and Rome (Fischer, 1996a, p. 26) (Figure 9.3):

> For if a man be placed flat on his back, with his hands and feet extended, and a pair of compasses entered at his navel, the fingers and toes of his two hands and feet will touch the circumference of a circle described there from. And just as the human body yields a circular outline, so, too, a square figure may be found from it. For if we measure the distance from the soles of the feet to the top of the head, and then apply that measure to the outstretched arms, the breadth will be found to be the same as the height, as in the case of plane surfaces which are perfectly square….The circumference of the circle is approximately equal to the periphery of the square
>
> *Vetruvius*

"Squaring the Circle," an archetypal idea from the mystery schools of Egypt, was based on shapes considered perfect and sacred. The circle represents a symbol of heavenly orbits while the square depicts the "foursquare" firmness of the earth. Placing a body image into the center of the superimposed shapes depicts a metaphor for unity of inner and outer worlds within the human being (Godwin, 1979).

Another Renisaissance painter, Albrecht Curer, included the use of harmonic scales (Fischer, 1996b, p. 37, 51) showing that the root harmonies of music, in keeping with Pythagorean concepts, correspond to good proportions in the human body. The idea of a correspondence between beauty as seen by the eye and harmony as heard by the ear begins to take on mystical proportions. Its relationship can be mathematically reproduced (Doczi, 1994, pp. 100–101) (Figure 9.4):

All parts of the human body share the same proportional limitations. The starting point unfolds at the center on top of the sacrum.

FIGURE 9.3

Human Form

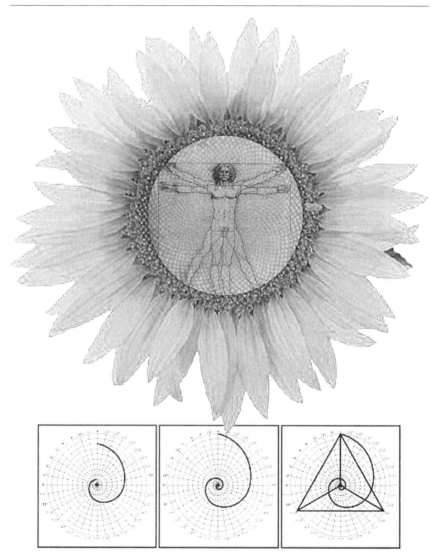

Because of its central location in the body, the length of the top half and bottom half of the body are similar. The hand is a microcosmic mirror of the body, growing out of the wrist as the spine grows out of the sacrum. The relationship between hand to arm to trunk

FIGURE 9.4

Human Form and Scale

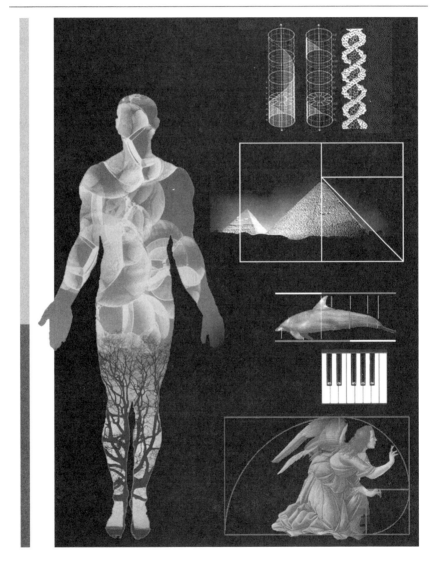

is also proportional, as is head to neck, trunk, legs, and feet. The graph illustrates the spread of approximations of human proportion to root harmonies found in music. Depicted are beautiful examples of proportional harmonies found throughout the body, demonstrating that we have a harmonious presence in the universe.

A Like a poised ballet dancer, our physical balancing center is located at the sacrum, while our spiritual center lies deep within our "human essence." The potential for harmony and beauty exists within each person. The potential for disease and disorder is also possible.

The expert nurse can sense subtle shifts in delicate balance, hear a misalignment in the symphonic sounds of body breath, a disrupted rhythm of circulation. Before heralding signs are measurable, this artist senses a shift below the obvious, hears the unspoken against a background of silence, noting an asymmetrical shift from the normal patterns of health.

As well as its basic contribution to formation of pattern, the harmonies and rhythms of dinergy also form the basis for sharing; the art of living. Sharing is a condition of life, a generous act of grace that unites diversity in life-giving ways. Light, color, and sound, the artist's tools, share the same wave patterns and the same vibrational rates. The essence of all vibration and rhythm is a harmonious sharing of diversities—weak and strong, in and out, up and down, back and forth—at reoccurring time intervals. This oscillating pattern occurs in the tide of the ocean, in our heartbeats, in the creation of light and sound, in the growth of a plant.

Dancers share information, energy and excitement, while friends share joys and concerns of the day. Shared stories and ideas in conversation, shared musical creation in song, shared worship in prayer, shared efforts toward problem resolution in community affairs, are part of everyday experience. The pattern of sharing is consistent in the birth of a phenomenon as well as throughout its dynamic growth and ultimate death. It emerges from a grateful heart. Albert Einstein observed that, "A hundred times every day I remind myself that my inner and outer life depend on the labors of other men, living and dead, and that I must exert myself in order to give in the same measure as I have received and am still receiving" (Einstein, 1953, p. 1).

Many animal species model sharing in each other's distress while rescuing endangered community members. Biologist Edward Wilson noted that mutual aid and cooperation were an essential part of evolution, a precursor to all moral behavior (Wilson, 2003); sharing is creative. As we share with those who have less, we acquire more than if we had kept all the resources to ourselves.

Unfortunately, the materialistic drive in contemporary society finds the line between competition and shared cooperation sometimes difficult to distinguish. In terms of current economic and political policy economist Barbara Ward observed, "When men or governments work intelligently and farsightedly for the good of others, they achieve their prosperity too....generosity is the best policy....our morals and our interest—seen in true perspective—do not pull us apart (Ward, 1992, p. 150)." Sharing as a basic pattern-forming process. It creates cooperation and abundance within a body, a group, and a civilization.

EXPANSION—THE ART OF LIVING

Our continued development as a human species, and as a universe, is toward increasing capacity for goodness coupled with an innate drive for increasing intelligence; a journey toward beauty and wisdom. "Beauty is the harmony and concord of all parts, achieved in such a manner that nothing could be added or taken away or altered except for the worse (Wittkower, 1992, p. 33)." History is filled with examples of too much leisure or luxury destroying our native beauty as well as it being destroyed by lack of life's basic necessities. Plato stated in his *Symposium*, that harmony and grace are born from the marriage of plenty and poverty. The pattern of sharing is a strong foundation that supports that which is beautiful and true to thrive in the world.

Our journey toward understanding is progressive, moving toward deeper "ways of knowing." We begin as children with the accumulation of facts and data. School fills us with information designed to give us a basic understanding of the world in which we live. As we age, life experience becomes the teacher. An encounter with reality gives us lessons that go beyond what can be found in a book. We may get misinformation, but we do not have a mis-experience. At some point in life, our worldview broadens and we begin to acquire knowledge, leading toward wisdom (Ardagh, 2005).

Ways of knowing are the keys to turning mere survival into the art of living. Knowledge, like science, is a logical taking apart, while wisdom, a form of art, is an intuitive putting together.... it synthesizes and integrates while knowledge analyzes and differentiates. Wisdom sees with eyes of mind, envisioning relation, wholeness and unity. Knowledge accepts what can be verified by the senses, grasping the specific and the diverse. Both wisdom and knowledge are based on experience, but knowledge retains experience through the filter of conceptual thought while wisdom speaks in images, symbols and paradox. These two diversities complement each other in dynergistic style.

However, there are times when things come into our lives that do not fit any of the categories of thought; it is the presence of mystery. It can be a profound and disrupting experience such as illness, death, a sudden unplanned change. At other times, numinous feelings can arise from a simple, daily observation made with sacred eyes. It can emerge from "seeing" the perfect pattern of wholeness in a flower, "smelling" the air after a spring rain, or "touching" someone we love. In these extra-ordinary moments we converge with the hidden, harmonious nature that unites us as a universal family. In that space lays the possibility for expanding our awareness and consciousness.

When we share our own specific limitations with those of others in dynergistic fashion, we compliment each other's shortcomings and emerge a stronger, larger whole of higher order. As an artist composing a life, we create living harmony comparable to the harmony found in the arts; music, dance, literature, and the sculpting of marble, wood, and clay.

Living in this fashion is our birthright; because nature's golden mean is part of the very fabric of our existence. The best human creations are timeless, ageless and holy. They are beautiful and harmonious, and graciously generous. As we live in harmony with All That Is, we step into alignment with the flow of life in all of nature, and we are at one.

> The only hope Mother Earth has for survival is our recovering creativity—
>> which is of course, our divine power.
>> Creativity is so satisfying, so important, not because it produces something but because the process is cosmological.
>> There's joy and delight in giving birth.
>
> Matthew Fox

Applying the Concepts in Nursing

Living a life of creative artistic expression means existing in the moment: being present with all of your senses to appreciate and savor the subtle in a material world. Ralph Waldo Emerson observed that "the invariable mark of wisdom is to see the miraculous in the common" (Shlain, 1991, p. 25).

The present moment is composed of the following qualities:

- *Alertness*: Being awake
- *Openness*: Being free from expectations
- *Freshness*: Not being overshadowed by the past
- *Innocence*: Not judging from old experiences
- *Spontaneity*: Allowing new impulses to come in without criticism or censorship
- *Fearlessness*: Absence of traumas from the past
- *Replenishing*: Capacity to renew oneself from within

All of these qualities are inherent in every human being; young children display them all of the time. You do not need to learn how to "be" these qualities—you must simply uncover and remember them into your life.

Checking In

A major block to recovering your innate capacity for "awe and wonder" is your tolerance level for uncertainty. As change accelerates in the world, we find that ambiguity is multiplying and things are less certain. The ability to embrace and thrive with ambiguity is the hallmark of a creative life.

Ambiguity Self-Assessment

- I am comfortable with ambiguity.
- I am attuned to the rhythms of my intuition.
- I thrive with change.
- I see the humor in life every day.
- I have the tendency to "jump to conclusions."
- I enjoy riddles, puzzles, and puns.
- I usually know when I am feeling anxious.
- I spend sufficient time on my own.
- I trust my gut.
- I can comfortably hold contradictory ideas in my mind.
- I delight in paradox and am sensitive to irony.
- I appreciate the importance of conflict in inspiring creativity.

Ambiguity can be a blessing when framed as such. Paradox teaches that ambiguity is the other side of curiosity, and the tension between these two poles fosters creativity. To make friends with ambiguity cultivate the capacity for confusion endurance. Balance will find you standing at the center of a unique Universe filled with paradox.

- *Joy and Sorrow*: What have been the saddest and happiest moments in your life? Do you ever feel both states simultaneously? "the highest happiness becomes the cause of future unhappiness...." Leonardo da Vinci
- *Intimacy and Independence*: Can you have one without the other? How does this play out in your most intimate relationships? Does this connection ever create anxiety?
- *Strength and Weakness*: Identify your three greatest strengths and your three greatest weaknesses. How are the qualities between them related?
- *Change and Constancy*: Identify three things that have remained consistent throughout your life, and three huge changes. Does the idea that "the more things change, the more they stay the same" have merit?
- *Humility and Pride*: What was the proudest moment of your life? When have you had your most profound feeling of genuine humility? How are these feelings different? Are there any unexpected similarities or are they total opposites?
- *Goals and Process*: Remember an important goal you established and the process utilized to get there. Have you ever achieved success without experiencing fulfillment? How do goal and process, doing and being relate?
- *Life and Death*: It is the tension between these two polarities that creates meaning in your life.

By facing these paradox and embracing the creative tension they stir, you will find magic in each day, just waiting for your artistic touch to bring it into manifestation (Gelb, 2000, pp. 154–155).

A Living Example

Distortions in art often make it easier for us to decipher what we are looking at especially when done by a master. Studies confirm that we are able to recognize visual exaggerations of distinct physical features in the drawing of a person, like a cartoon portrait of George Bush or Richard Nixon more quickly than an actual photo.

Famous cubist artist Pablo Picasso observed that art is the lie that reveals the truth. In 1906, Picasso decided to reinvent the boundaries of portrait painting, pushing the boundaries of realism. Rather than carefully reflecting what was in front of him, he decided to capture the essence of his subject, Gertrude Stein, in a new way. For months he struggled in his Paris studio, never satisfied with his work. Then he went on a trip to Spain; it changed his life and his work forever.

While traveling in Spain he studied the people and landscape with an open and questioning mind. With fresh eyes he saw the weathered face of the Spanish peasants, the ancient art of Iberia. Upon returning to Paris, he took a whole new approach to portrait painting. He gave Ms. Stein's portrait the head of a primitive mask, flattening her face and depicting it with a series of dramatic angles. Picasso intentionally exaggerated prominent aspects of her appearance. He focused on the most distinctive features of her face; heavy, lidded eyes and long, aquiline nose, overstating them in angular fashion. Despite the artistic license, the painting is still recognizable as Stein. Through careful distortion, he found a way to intensify reality. This became the foundation of his life as a cubist artist.

Scientific studies show that the brain recognizes specific prominent facial features to distinguish one face from another. The fusiform gyrus, the area of the brain involved in facial recognition, responds more quickly to caricatures than to real faces because those features are more highly exaggerated. Abstractions, like the art work of Picasso, act as a super-stimulus and foster a peak-shift in brain recognition. Art, in the end, lies in the eyes of the beholder. So what do you depict in your life which is a work of art? (http://www.psychologytoday.com/articles/200907/unlocking-the-mysteries-the-artistic-mind)

Web Site Resource: Becoming an artist means reinventing yourself through mindful creativity. To explore your abilities and interests in a creative approach to life, you may wish to explore the following Web site and others like it:

http://www.wikihow.com/Become-an-Artist

BIBLIOGRAPHY

Abram, D. (1996). *The spell of the sensuous: Perception and language in a more-than-human world*. New York, NY: Pantheon Books.

Anodea, J. (2004). *Eastern body, western mind*. Berkley, CA: Celestial Arts.

Ardagh, A. (2005). *The translucent revolution*. Novato, CA: New World Press.

Doczi, G. (1994). *The power of limits: Proportional harmonies in nature, art and architecture*. Boston, MA: Shambhala Publications.

Dowson, R. (1979). *Art in its own terms*. New York, NY: Taplinger.

Einstein, A. (1953). *The world as i see it*. New York, NY: Oxford University Press.

Fischer, B. (1996a). *Man, grand reflection of the greater cosmos: Occult Anatomy* (Vol. 1). Prescott, AZ: Subru Publications.

Fischer, B. (1996b). *Pythagorean numerology: A summary of the esoteric properties of numbers*. Prescott, AZ: Clarity Works.

Gelb, M. (2000). *How to think like Leonardo da Vinci: Seven steps to genius every day*. New York, NY: Dell Press.

Godwin, J. (1979). *Robert Fludd*. Boulder, CO: Shambhala Publications.

Chipp, H. B. (1956). *Theories of modern art*. Berkley, CA: University of California Press.

Kaku, M. (1994). *Hyperspace: A Scientific Odyssey through parallel universes, time warps, and the 10th dimension*. New York, NY: Doubleday.

Leshan, L., & Margenau, H. (1982). *Einstein's space & Van Gogh's sky: Physical reality and beyond*. New York, NY: Macmillan Publishing Company.

Malcolm, P. (1994). *Evolution of the soul*. Victoria, Australia: Inward Path Publishers.

Pesut, D., & Herman, J. A. (1999). *Clinical reasoning: The art & science of critical & creative thinking*. Boston, MA: Delmar Publishing.

Reed, L. (1968). *Art now*. London, UK: Faber & Faber.

Shlain, L. (1991). *Art & physics: Parallel visions in space, time & light*. New York, NY: Quill Publishing Company.

Steiner, R. (2001). *The fourth dimension: Sacred geometry, alchemy and mathematics*. Great Barrington, MA: Anthroposophic Press.

Ward, B. (1992). *The rich nations and the poor nations*. New York, NY: W.W. Norton.

Wilson, E. (2003). *The future of life*. New York, NY: Random House Press.

Wittkower, R. (1992). *Architectural principles in the age of humanism*. London, UK: Alec Tiranti.

CHAPTER 10

THE HUMAN SPIRIT
UNFOLDING INNER POTENTIAL

*Within each individual on this large and complicated world there lives
an astonishing potential of greatness. Yet it is rare that these hidden gifts are
brought to life unless by chance of fate or commitment to inner growth.*

Unknown Teacher

We stand poised on the threshold of human history where
humanity is on the brink of a new understanding regarding
the true depth of our human potential. The ongoing saga of war
and terrorism reminds us of the depths to which we can plunge
when fear and anger rule. At the same time, we see reflections
of the best of human nature in the demonstrated love and hero-
ism that depicts a greater humanity. Nowhere is this more evident
than in the practice of nursing.

Lakota spiritual teacher Wanigi Waci teaches that the antidote
to war is service. Because everything in the universe is in a state of
dynamic balance, for everyone engaged in war and killing there is
one who is being supported in suffering, and nursing (offered by
professional nurses and lay people who support their loved ones)
is holding the world in balance. He also believes that peace and
global unity will not come about through economic development.
Rather, they will come about through professional nursing, the largest tribe of feminine energy globally. He believes that nurse migra-
tion will be the vehicle for unification of humanity. Nurses who
migrate have a spirit of adventure, courage, and compassion. They
will move into other parts of the world and marry into the predominant culture. Their offspring will be multiracial, adventuresome,
courageous, and compassionate, and they will be the seed crystals
of a new race that will unify the globe in a spirit of love and service.

275

As his story illustrates, we can explore the rich journey of the universe across time from multiple perspectives including science, religion, philosophy, literature, and the arts. Walking with our ancestors, we see the result of forces acting upon them many millennia ago. What becomes clear is the fact that what we will be tomorrow depends on our present choices, choices strongly influenced by a number of constraints that are part of the evolutionary makeup of humanity.

Our unfolding story is influenced by the genes that make up the human body, by instincts that trigger an action below the level of conscious awareness. Choices are strongly influenced by cultural heritage, the systems that code "appropriate" behavior, often limiting us to conduct better suited to some past time. And then there is the belief system of religion that fosters intolerance of others who are not "members." Recognition of the forces and choices that limit our journey toward increasing consciousness and human capacity makes it possible to become liberated from them (Ardaga, 2005).

A new urgency is felt in our continuing search for self-awareness. For the past 400 years, the world of science has given us discoveries that would have amazed our ancestors. It has explained the birth of the universe from a tiny seed to a self-expanding cosmos and provided images of immense galaxies and subatomic quarks. However, science alone cannot provide what we need today, for we are now moving beyond our physical existence in the external world into an equally daring and disciplined exploration of our inner life. The threshold we are crossing moves us into the landscape of the soul and transcendence, leading to personal and global transformation.

As we review the unfolding history of human potential, the evolution of human capacity from a tiny cell to spectacular new abilities and levels of experience becomes evident. Humankind's exploration of the inner life is uncovering new frontiers of creativity, which are antidotes for the hatred and alienation that have plagued us for so long. It heralds the dawn of a cultural transformation beyond anything we have heretofore imagined.

OUR BEGINNINGS—A SLOW AND SOLITARY JOURNEY

In his compelling book, *A Brief History of Everything*, Ken Wilbur observes that "There is a common evolutionary thread running from matter to life to mind. Certain common patterns, or laws, or habits keep repeating themselves in all those domains (Wilber, 1996)." He suggests that, according to the world's great wisdom traditions, looking at those extraordinary patterns reveals the unfolding of *Spirit in action*. Every stage of development finds consciousness manifesting and realizing more of itself, recognizing more of its own true nature.

Stages of higher development modeled by ancient teachers and adepts reflect our own deep potential. Looking carefully at these lives in light of our own continuing emergence informs us about what personal and collective evolution has in store for us tomorrow. This helps us make concrete sense of the experiences and observations that comprise our own path toward wholeness. As we identify and practice new ways of being, we are transformed.

Great debate exists within the scientific, philosophical, and religious worlds regarding the theory of evolution. The facts demonstrating our continuing development and advancement as a universe, a civilization, as individuals are everywhere noted (Berry & Swimme, 1992; Kaufman, 1995; Lloyd, 1923; Rifkin, 2009). In spite of growing evidence, some people still deny its existence. "One cause of such misunderstanding is a failure to distinguish evolution as fact from theories on how and why it is happening" (Redfield & Murphy, 2002, p. 73).

However explained and understood, the meandering course of evolution from the beginning of the universe, to the appearance of living species, and the emergence of humanity has created the inorganic, biological, and human worlds. In this pattern, we can see that even the process of evolution has evolved. The underlying pattern of this ever-evolving universe is movement to ever greater complexities in the material world and the growing capacities of humanity.

The appearance of plant life and the emergence of humanity marked the beginnings of two new evolution eras; these were moments of evolutionary transcendence (Pearce, 2002). Quantum shifts of this magnitude were made possible through the countless changes in complexity that preceded them. Evolutionary theorist Stebbins (1969) noted that approximately 640,000 small steps in organic evolution resulted in less than 100 major changes in plant and animal development during hundreds of millions of years of evolutionary progress.

Humankind has followed the same prefigured design in our development across time. Patterns and trends suggest that we are approaching an emerging evolutionary domain similar to the epic shift from inorganic to plant life or the emergence of human form. The convergence of the birth of spiritual awareness among our ancestors and the recent scientific discoveries about the untapped capacities for life are potentiating a shift of unprecedented nature.

Evolution began accelerating our human journey with the convergence of intelligence, communication, and domestic skills. Our species began to form creative social groups, harness fire, develop tools, form words, communicate, and create art forms. In the Stone Age, our evolutionary journey was launched as we continued our efforts to make sense of the world in which we live.

At one point these ancestors began to develop markedly beyond the capacity of their forbearers. *Shamans* were centrally involved in this acceleration of human development in various roles such as medicine men and women, masters of ritual, artists, and guides to worlds beyond the senses. Shamans have long been the primary mediators within their communities while also offering contact with the spirit world. Although they were expert at healing and assisting with love and battle, their greatest contribution was in their capacity for altered states of consciousness used in healing, dream interpretation, and bringing the community closer to other worlds.

Studies in the Americas, Siberia, Central Asia, and Australia show remarkable similarities between shamanic practices worldwide. Most Stone-Age cultures believed that a shaman in trance would transverse other worlds to assist with their activities around healing physical and spiritual ailments and better preside over rites of passage such as marriage, birth and death. Shamanism was the first institutionalization of visions and practices that opened extraordinary powers to contact the Transcendent. They were the forerunners of the prophets, saints, and seers of the world's great religions (Harner, 1990).

SHARING THE PATH—A CONVERGENCE OF COLLECTIVES

Thousands of years after the appearance of shamanism, the birth of *mystery schools* appeared in Greece, Syria, Anatolia, Egypt, and Persia. They involved similar activities including adoration of a specific deity, rites of spiritual transformation, and very elaborate religious rituals and dramas. These rituals and teachings fostered an intuitive sense that the soul is secretly connected with the divine, pointing countless people toward a greater life to come (Hall, 1986; Meyer, 1987)

During the second millennia B.C.E., another significant step in human consciousness occurred in India with the emergence of the *Vedic* culture. The oldest collection of religious texts used today, they are divided into four bodies: hymns, prayers, rites, and healing practices; mythologies of ancient India; spiritual philosophy; and instructions for yoga practices. These were developed to put these teachings into the hands of the people, literally allowing them to "sit at the feet of the masters" (Pannikar, 1977).

Between the 7th and 4th century B.C.E. in the Middle East, Asia, and Greece, another spiritual awakening occurred, referred to as "*the Axial Age*" because of its impact on people living in one half of the world. China experienced the emergence of Taoism while Greece and Athens experienced the awakening of philosophy. The Jews were guided by great prophets, while India was incorporating the teachings of Buddha. The countless insights from this era seeded the beginnings of the evolutionary leap we are about to take today.

The *Tao Te Ching*, written by Lao-Tze in the 6th century B.C.E., articulated the convergence of Chinese philosophy and shamanism. It gave rise to: metaphysical teachings; the practice of feng shui, which helps landscaping lie in accord with natural contours and forces; calligraphy, which calls for the student to trust the hand's instinctive flow; acupuncture, herbal medicines, and tai chi, all of which are based on movements that harmonize the body with the energy of *chi*; and Taoist art, including the yin-yang symbol widely used today. More than any sacred tradition before or since, Taoism supports a philosophy and set of practices that promote aesthetic harmony with all that is (Lao-Tzu, 1992, 2001).

In the 5th century B.C.E., *Buddhism* was the reforming religious culture in India, which remains the primary laboratory and disseminator of this philosophy today. Gautama Buddha, the founder, identified "four noble truths." The first states that all life is marked by suffering; the second notes that suffering is caused by desire; the third states that there is release from suffering by "blowing out" the flames of desire; and, the fourth highlights the way to nirvana via the "eightfold noble path." This path includes right understanding, right thought, right speech, right action, right livelihood, right effort, right concentration, and right mindfulness (Armstrong, 2001).

This spiritual tradition stresses commitment to ideas and the practice of disciplines that can produce freedom from suffering while promoting spiritual understanding through detachment and the acquisition of wisdom. A primary tenet of the belief system is a powerful ethic of service to those in need. The spirit of compassion is accentuated in the doctrine of the bodhisattva. Within this tradition is a vast information store regarding human development that is essential as the world becomes increasingly complex. Its power lies in the integration of Taoist, Shaman, Zen, and other practices into its roots within the yogas of ancient India (Hahn, 1999).

In making these cultural adaptations, Buddhism has transcended the insights of its founder and early practitioners, becoming a great repository of liberating practices that can transform our potential including meditation, visualization, energy mobilization, mindfulness training. Its greatest power lies in its learned ability to adapt these transformative disciplines to the various cultures in order to enhance their adoption. As we move more toward our emergent nature, our understanding will increasingly incorporate some of these practices.

While the East was moving in this direction, Greek city-states began to emerge on the Mediterranean Sea. The seeds of Western culture were planted; with developments in mathematics and discoveries in the physical world, with the unfolding of rhetoric and philosophy, with a blending of history, art and politics that gave rise to individual rights.

One of Greece's greatest gifts however, was fostered with the presence of Plato and Socrates. These physically and spiritually vigorous men, through their *philosophical dialogue* and *rhetoric,* gave birth to the capacity for self-reflection and self-understanding. Living from 470 to 399 B.C.E., Socrates, was a prominent critic of conventional opinion. His liberating skepticism questioned conventional assumptions about the world, and he declared that the unexamined life was not worth living (Guthrie, 1960). He stimulated self-inquiry, examination of social norms, and established the "Socratic method" of inquiry that has inspired ethical integrity for several millennia.

His famous student, Plato, became a great philosopher who explored timeless questions regarding identity and the ways we acquire knowledge. He examined practical ways to live a good life, improve education and social politics. He founded "The Academy" on his family's land, which flourished for 900 years. At this place, students were guided to find the true, the good, and the beautiful through practiced acts of contemplation, discourse, and moral behavior.

Both men brought an unprecedented intellectual range and flexibility, integrating the physical, social, moral, and spiritual worlds of their time. Aristotle, Plato's greatest student, took their work to another level when he developed his Theory of Forms, holding that eternal ideas corresponded with humanities less than perfect efforts. He was the founder of classification systems, setting standards that later established the field of biology. His work would be pivotal in guiding Charles Darwin's evolutionary theory many years later.

The cumulative work of these early intellectual explorers influenced subsequent Jewish, Christian, and Islamic philosophy and practice. These *courageous pioneers of the integral spirit* showed the world how to combine seemingly unrelated functions of social understanding, philosophical speculation, mystical insight, and the individual practice of virtue. Their playful, fertile, and creative experimentation laid the groundwork for the intellectual flexibility and individual morality of future generations, including our own (Plato, 1928).

The Axial Age was also influenced by the great *Jewish Prophets*, Isaiah, Micah, Amos, Jeremiah, and Elijah, who lived between the 9th and 4th centuries B.C.E. They broadened the tribal view of Yahweh, making him a God for all people. They reinforced the notion that all men and women, including the sick and disadvantaged, were equally children of this Living God. They underscored the need for ethical standards if people are to live peacefully together. In addition, they set the stage for religion to become a strong political force (Heschel, 1956).

One of the greatest contributions of the Jewish age was their emphasis on life as a journey toward better things. It was a sharp break from the cyclical nature of life as proposed by Eastern and Greek belief systems. Jewish life was viewed as a mystical practice leading toward union with God. Such a life required social justice and nonviolence, universal love and forgiveness, and a life of active service to the less fortunate. Many of these tenets would later influence Martin Buber (1878–1965) and other contemporary psychologists.

Several centuries later, another Jewish prophet emerged, Jesus of Nazareth. Six hundred years before he appeared, the Jews had begun to look for a Messiah; many inside and outside of the Jewish faith identified him as the One. Within 300 years of Jesus death, *Christianity* had become the dominant religion of the Roman Empire, and in the two millennia since, it has become the most popular religion on earth. The principal message of this belief system is the necessity of letting God's love for humanity flow from ourselves to others, even those who attack us. It is a message of unconditional love, Christian fellowship with others, and a life of compassion, forgiveness, and service. By embodying Jesus' teaching that God's love channeled through us can save the world, we develop our capacities for transformation and further spiritual advance (Stephen, 1999).

Islam is the second most popular and the fastest growing world religion today. With roots in Abraham, it moved through Judaism and Christianity, only to be redefined by Muhammad who felt the message was too distorted. Devotional practices, including prayer 5 times daily, demonstrate a commitment to God. Three blessings are given, thru *Sufism*, to those who love God with devotion; submission, faith, and an abiding awareness of God. The quest for a direct experience of God is both the crown of religious life and the path toward truth (Nicholson, 1967).

Since the mid-20th century, Sufism has been growing in Europe and America amongst people seeking authentic spiritual realization that transcends monasticism. Many teachers, such as Gurdjieff (Fisher, 1996), have inspired groups devoted to meditation, self-inquiry, and devotional exercises developed in esoteric Sufi schools. Though Islam, like many religions, has bred dogmatism and intolerance, it also has elevated the moral and spiritual lives of people worldwide.

Expanding Understanding—Movement From Religious to Secular

The movement of the *Renaissance* flourished during Europe's Middle Ages. This period of rebirth was a precursor to the Modern Age. An era of unprecedented development spanned the arenas of art and science, religion and philosophy, architecture and social systems. However, it did not resolve the great suffering of the masses, as war and poverty spawned by the Crusades and the decline of the Greco-Roman empire continued a caste system of government (Tarnas, 1991).

Leonardo Da Vinci embodied the ideal Renaissance personality; a self-described "disciple of experiment." His work was infused with great originality that focused on problems of science and society, with notable outcomes in the design of buildings and machines, weapons of war, and works of art. Simultaneously, as great scientists and artists creativity overflowed, the turning toward supernatural beliefs of the past era was increasingly reinforced by the worldly realism of emerging science and the affirmation of the individual. The Renaissance was an era whose emphasis was on human expression, power and fulfillment, and the embracing of discoveries, inventions, and insights birthed in an atmosphere committed to the love of learning and creativity (Leonardo Da Vinci, 1956).

As the 18th century began, the focus on man and nature had moved Westward. It was kindled by freedom of expression with speech and pen. Increasingly frequent and direct communication, coupled with the use of reason, and a revolt against religious oppression or the rule of kings, fostered stunning advances in science and technology. Those seeking "truth" were searching for a clarifying and unifying vision to transcend the destructive religious conflicts of the day. This quest gave birth to the *Scientific Revolution and the Enlightenment.*

In the light of increasing scientific discovery, supernatural explanations were no longer needed to explain the world and human nature. The ensuing literary, scientific, and philosophical movements amongst notables such as Copernicus, Galileo, Newton, and other scientists, along with Descartes, Locke and Hume and other thinkers, built on their rich past while challenging traditional wisdom. The call went out for intellectual liberty, the emergence of reason, and the testing and validating of the irrefutable laws of science (Kuhn, 1970).

While science was progressive, its shadow side began to emerge. Scientists increasingly rejected the findings of contemplatives as science increasingly turning away from confirmable facts of the inner life. Many also began to reject all spiritual phenomena, giving rise to a strictly materialistic view of the world and humankind. Along with the liberation of the human spirit and overthrow of despotic regimes, the use and abuse of science also contributing to the exploitation and destruction of the earth and the natural world—a trend that continues today.

As we review the great human journey, the story reveals a greater life pressing to be born within humanity. We see that as certain practices are incorporated into daily life, enlarging capacities can be nurtured and eventually integrated as a permanent aspect of our being. We also develop an appreciation for the fundamental social forces that work against them.

As people, we are seeking for a worldview that gives both context and guidance to our quest to transcend the dogma and superstition that has for so long divided us. Contemporary spiritual leaders such as Vietnamese Buddhist monk Thich Nhat Hahn have observed that the next Buddha will not appear in the form of an individual. Instead, the new spiritually centered force will emerge in the form of a community of people living in loving kindness and mindful awareness (Pearce, 2004). Nursing holds the potential for serving society in this capacity today.

THE POSSIBLE HUMAN—A BIOLOGY OF TRANSCENDENCE

Since the beginning of the early 19th century, both scholars and scientists have unearthed a wide range of discoveries to create the largest body of knowledge ever available on the extraordinary capacity of human functioning. Coupled with increasing access to wisdom literature translated into multiple languages, there has emerged a vast array of educational and therapeutic experiments, and countless empirical studies on human capacity, the range and creativity that is breathtaking in its scope.

Transcendence implies the ability to rise above and move beyond. There is a bitter irony in the fact that we have a history so rich in lofty philosophy and noble ideas, and yet are experiencing a degree of violence unprecedented in human history. New studies demonstrate that neither our violence nor our capacity for transcendence is specifically a moral/ethical issue. Rather, it is primarily a biological one (Pearce, pp. 27–32).

Our history of behavior has derailed our personal development of biological capacities for transcendence. We continue to project the "bad" that is out there toward each other, while the "good" is transferred to the wise and sage amongst us. A new breed of biologists and neuroscientists has uncovered the root to our paradoxical behavior of feeling one thing, saying another, and acting from an impulse different from either.

These new scientists have discovered that we have five different neural structures, or brains, within us. Four of the five lie within our head, representing the whole evolution of life preceding us: reptilian, old mammalian, new mammalian and human. Each new structure emerged to offer us the possibility of "going beyond" former behavior, while simultaneously creating new problems for us to solve.

The fifth brain of our system lies in our heart, just as poets have long believed. The new field of neurocardiology has uncovered this brain center in our heart, which functions in a dynamic way with the fourfold brain in our head. This head–heart dynamic affects, reflects, and determines our responsiveness outside the field of our conscious awareness. As we become more aware of nature's head–heart dynamic, we begin to cooperate with this mutually interdependent spirit and the collaborative activity between our intelligence and our intellect, our biology and our spirit. The unification and transcendence of our splintered selves may be the next intelligent evolutionary shift.

The path-breaking studies of leading neuroscientist Paul MacLean, span more than 6 decades, and give a clear map of three neural systems in our head and the parallel connection to three major evolutionary periods in the universe, reptilian, old mammalian, and new mammalian. Each neural system carries a blueprint of potential intelligences, abilities and capabilities developed during each epoch (MacLean, 1993).

Nature never abandons a working system, but instead enlarges and expands the old to increase efficiency. Each new evolutionary brain was established to solve a challenge in our ever-changing environment. When each gets integrated into the other our capacity increases tenfold. However, when integration fails, we become a house divided against itself, with great inner (and outer) conflict the result.

Our *hindbrain*, the reptilian brain, is the oldest member whose primary function is giving us awareness of the outer sensory world. Comprised of the sensory-motor system, the spinal cord and vast network of neural connections, this process functions well below our level of awareness. It manages our physical well-being by controlling basic physiological activity. It functions in a very habitual, patterned way and cannot alter its inherited or learned patterns of behavior.

Originally designed to elude predators, this oldest structure is highly skilled at deceptive procedures. It helps us to be multifaceted when threatened, and can be used, in conjunction with our higher neocortex, to rationalize and justify morally deceptive behavior.

This brain registers present tense only. In emergencies, its reflexive system can alert the neocortex to mobilize all systems for body defense. Emotion has no impact on this center, so clarity and swiftness are its hallmarks. However, there is an interpreter mode between this brain and the neocortex that passes through our emotional-cognitive system upon command. This broader connection allows for the neocortex to stand back and moderate or redirect a sensory report, minimizing what at times could be a violent reaction from the predatory nature of this brain center.

The second brain to emerge in humankind was the old mammalian, *limbic,* or emotional-cognitive brain. Here nature added to the limited reptilian senses the extraordinary senses of smell and hearing, which opened up a whole new world of higher order for the sensory system. As the seat of learning and memory, this space is encoded with multiple functions and behaviors, which includes a mothering capacity to serve as the limbic function for an infant until this aspect of its brain is fully developed at the age of three.

This nurturing emotional brain computes a past and present state and serves as the foundation for relationships. It gives us an awareness of our interior subjective world along with our feelings concerning the outer world and our relationship with it. Emotions are the collective tools we use to qualitatively evaluate our relationships, facilitating an association to the world as a sophisticated object standing "outside" of it, rather than from a simple reflexive act.

The newer mammalian brain, or *neocortex*, serves as our verbal-intellectual brain. This brain possesses the awareness of past, present and future. It introduces language and thinking, the capacity to observe all factors in a situation rather than react from instinct alone. This high brain is 5 times larger than the other two combined, hosting a hundred billion neurons, each capable of interacting with a hundred thousand others to create fields of coordinated action. Neural fields constantly shift and change to update their intelligence reports, translating external information and data into thought and imagination within.

Evolution opened an entirely new universe with the gift of awareness embedded in the neocortex. With a capacity to predict the future, problem solving became a human potential. The high brain also holds an impulse toward novelty that fosters creative imagination, our highest human capacity (Steiner, 1969).

Brain development occurs in a nested hierarchy, beginning with reptilian brain in the first trimester of pregnancy, followed by the old mammalian in the second trimester and the human brain in the third. A new fourth brain makes its entrance after birth. What makes each of these evolving neural systems uniquely human is the overall context into which they are placed, each articulating with the other while holding limitless capacity for network development with similar fields.

Bruce Lipton, cellular biologist, (Lipton & Bertsch, 1991) demonstrated how the first cell created is a template for all subsequent cellular development. The essential nature of any old system is that it maintains its integrity while playing a new and expanded role in partnership with emerging new structures. In a two-way exchange, each cell and each brain modifies the other to some degree. The resulting movement beyond limitations, the hallmark of transcendence, is not reached at the expense of any other system. This facilitates a sustaining field for all involved.

Whether we live a life of creative adventure or close ourselves in a defensive way depends to a large extent upon the first years of life when the new fourth brain, the *prefrontal cortex*, emerges to support our higher intellect (Ferris, 1992). This most recent and largest brain addition resides in the ridge of our brow. Functions attributed to it include the higher human virtues of love, compassion, empathy and understanding as well as advanced intellectual skills. It is considered to house the seat of higher intellect; our ability to compute, reason and analyze, and think creatively. It also includes our ability to regulate emotions, control our impulses, and modify reflexive behavior; in other words, it governs the activity of the other three brains in civilized fashion (Jerison, 1997).

Schore's prolific work in this area shows that development of the prefrontal lobes is experience-dependent; the environment must provide appropriate stimuli if full growth is to occur. First stage growth occurs within the first year of life, and again in mid-adolescence if adequate affirmation in a positive environment is experienced. Full development occurs around the age 21, with yet another chance for transcendence at approximately age 30 (Schore, 1994).

If life is filled with fear, violence, shaming, rules, and other emotionally depleting activities such as stress and anxiety within the mother or the environment, the prefrontal lobes decline. Nurturing an infant induces long lasting changes in the adult frontal cortex, leading to permanent modifications that increase exploratory behavior and playfulness, important roles in regulating higher-order information processing.

Failure to nurture leads to increasing inability of young people to modify primitive impulses and behaviors as this coordinating function is diminished. Statistics from 1995 indicate that on average, everyday in America, 18 children were shot by other children. As of 2000, suicide became the third leading cause of death in children between ages 5 and 17. Continued exposure to violence in music and film, guns and police protection in the school systems, terrorism in the news and an endless string of "no" and "don't" must be vigorously offset with an emphasis on the nurturance and love of infants and adolescents if this alarming trend is to be reversed (Pearce, 2004, p. 148).

Six decades ago cellular research led to the discovery that alters not only the way we view the heart but also our relationship to the universe. The discovery of the triune heart—electromagnetic, neural and hormonal in nature—fostered a new field of medicine, neurocardiology (Armour & Ardell, 1994). While all living forms produce an electrical charge, the heart cell has an electrical output 40 to 60 times greater than a brain wave. This energy forms an electromagnetic field that extends 12 to 15 feet beyond our body, its greatest strength residing in the first three feet.

The traditional view of the heart as a pump is enriched when examined from the perspective of the triune heart, where the pumping function is enhanced by the synchronistic contraction and expansion of the blood vessels themselves, the motility and plasticity of blood cells that change shape according to the size of vessel they are moving through, contraction of the skeletal muscles, and the flow of blood in spiral-like vortices from

FIGURE 10.1

The Heart's Torus

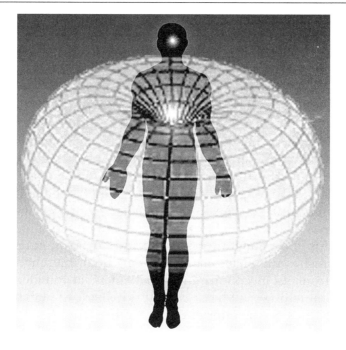

grooves built into the blood vessels themselves. As blood dashes into the heart chamber from an open heart valve, the rush of swirling blood forms a vortex, adding to its electromagnetic field (Marinelli, 1995) (Figure 10.1).

The force of this electromagnetic field produces a torus, much as magnets create an arc from filings placed within their field. The axis of this torus extends from the pelvic floor to the top of the skull. Comprised of an organic and living force, the torus is a very stable energy field that tends to self-perpetuate. Scientists conjecture that all energy systems, from the smallest atomic field to the largest universal level, are toroid in form. This leads to speculation that there is one universal torus that encompasses an infinite number of interacting, holographic tori within its spectrum (Childre, 1999).

Our solar system, with the sun at center, is also toroidal in nature. Fluctuations within its energy field impact all others through the corresponding magnetic lines of earth. We exist in a nested hierarchy of torid energy systems, making each of us as much the center of the universe as any other point or creature. Because these electromagnetic fields are holographic in nature, this gives us equal access to all that exists (Greene, 1999).

Producing energy is the first characteristic of the triune heart. Neurotransmitters, the second trait, create the "brain in the heart" as over half of the cardiac cells are comprised of neurons, clustered into ganglia similar to those found in the brain. One aggregate of the heart's neural ganglia is scattered throughout body tissue, muscle spindles, and organs through a connection to the spinal cord and peripheral neuron system. A second grouping has direct and unmediated connection with the emotional limbic brain, fostering an ongoing dialogue between heart and brain.

In embryonic and fetal development, a rudimentary human heart comes first, followed by the formation of brain, and then the body. Before becoming a four-chambered heart, the rudimentary heart furnishes the electromagnetic (em) field that envelops the embryo from its inception. This em field is surrounded by the mother's more powerful heart energy, stabilizing the infant's heart field as it takes on the imprint of the mother.

The third influencer of the heart on the brain is hormonal in nature, resulting in the conclusion that the heart is an endo-crine gland (Raloff, 1998). The atrium of the heart produces the hormone ANF, which can influence and modulate the emotional-cognitive system of the brain. Other heart-generated hormones have also been uncovered, including tranquilizers that keep us in balance and harmony with each other and the earth. Because the heart is connected to every facet of both the body and the brain, it is the intellect of the heart, not the brain that must coordinate the signals from the pancreas, liver, spleen, and so on.

The heart, earth, and sun provide the earth's electromag-netic spectrum, supplying the fundamental materials for creating our reality. Our heart's em field shields us from inappropriate fre-quencies while also selecting, from the larger hologram in which we are nested, frequency groupings that facilitate our growth, development and ongoing life. Through this holographic hierar-chy of em fields, we can modulate our heart and brain frequen-cies with those of the earth, creating a reciprocal relationship between us.

The heart and mind connection speaks through emotions. However, the heart has no neural structures to perceive or analyze the context, nature, details, or logic of our emotional reports. The heart is unable to judge the validity of these reports, so responds to them as basic facts. A state of harmony and love connects us to the high cortical areas where creativity and problem solving reside. If the message is negative, the heart makes an adaptive shift from the slower reflective intellect (slow thoughts) of the frontal lobes and neocortex to the swift reptilian brain (fast thoughts) linked with the emotional brain where survival memories and maneuvers reside.

This sudden shift from forebrain to hindbrain is not voluntary, it occurs outside of our awareness. In this archaic and defensive mindset, we have limited access to our intellectual capacity, falling back on our defenses or revenge strategies. These ancient patterns are supported by powerful field energies of consensual reality; group mindset and crowd comfort. These fields are constantly reinforced through much of the information and activity occurring in the mass culture in which we reside. We pick up that vibrational energy as surely as we respond to our own, unless there is a conscious effort to detach from it.

Our emerging potential cannot be utilized nor can our dilemma get resolved by intellect or ethical efforts alone. *The hope for transcendence lies in our ability to break from the mass mindset, and turn to our heart.* The minute we recognize that a stressful event is forming, we can shift our focus from the threat to our heart. Recalling an event infused with love and gratitude immediately blocks the automatic negative reaction to a stressful event. From this quiet and centered place, we can hear the wisdom of our heart and body-mind, selecting options that move toward our well-being as well as that of the world (40).

In his compelling work on an Empathic Civilization, Rifkin (2009) explores human history and the meaning of human existence in an alternative way. Rather than focusing on conflicts and power struggles, he examined human progress through the lens of empathic evolution. Empathy is viewed as active engagement where the observer is compelled to become part of another's experience; both joy and suffering. His research identifies a "Fourth Instinct"—the part of human character that compels us to go beyond our impulse for survival, sex, and power, driving us to expand the boundaries of our caring to include the communities and world around us. Rather than an isolated event that occurs in major crisis such as the earthquakes of Haiti, countless acts of empathic support are shown in relationships daily.

At specific times in human history, new energy regimes converge with new communication revolutions, creating more complex societies. The current technology explosion coupled with the World Wide Web has brought together more diverse people, heightening empathic sensitivity, which expands human consciousness. Ironically, the growing empathy requires ever-greater resource consumption, which negatively impacts the health of the planet. The challenge is to rise above the noise and clutter of our daily lives and engage the larger questions of life, expanding our economic, political, and relational models in a way that will bring empathy rather than greed into the choices we make. Our individual and collective choices, coupled with the morality of our leaders, will make the difference between destruction or healing of the world and everything on it.

At each moment we must open ourselves again and again, taking responsibility for making each decision consciously through our emerging new intelligence until, at last, we have shifted the focal point of our response to life into the transcendent realm of active intelligence. This begins our true healing journey.

> *Someday, after mastering winds, waves, tides and gravity,*
> *We shall harness the energy of love,*
> *And for the second time in the history of the world,*
> *Man will have discovered fire.*
>
> Pierre Teilhard De Chardin

Applying the Concepts in Nursing

A conscious life is a life of moral leadership. Rather than being a corporate position of influence, leadership is taking responsibility for living your life with such integrity and vision that others join you in making the world a better place. Sometimes you are the leader, at other times you follow respectfully. It is this iterative process that helps us become the master of our own destiny. Specific developmental tasks to be achieved at each stage of leadership are listed. A "Checking In" Quiz invites you to test your perception regarding what comprises the "developmental task" and how well you have accomplished it for yourself. It is important to note that a leadership style generates, and often is supported by, a corresponding followership style.

LEADERSHIP DEVELOPMENT ANALYSIS

Style 1: Autocratic Dictator Manager—The Controlling Stage

The beginning leader moves from fear and distrust toward a beginning sense of security through basic life-skill development.

Leadership Style

- Maintains physical and social distance from others
- Makes all major decisions alone
- Seeks to control as much as possible
- Demands loyalty to her/him as well as the unit/organization

Follower Behaviors

- Views the leader as distant and unapproachable
- Follows passively with blind obedience
- Sees the leader as having an aura of infallibility around him/her
- Demonstrates infantile type behavior

Characteristics of this Stage

Starting Point	Well Developed
Insecure and dependent	Secure and dependent
Isolated	Becoming connected
Uninformed	Seeking information
Helpless and hopeless	Helpful and hopeful

Impact of style on group/organization:

This style may be necessary in times of imminent danger. However, it becomes destructive when the environment is secure. Such a leader has difficulty delegating any activities that may diminish their power. This style is particularly distressful when the followers hold values on a more advanced level, experiencing the leader's style as oppressive and unjust.

Checking In: To what extent (on a scale of 1–5)

- Do you feel most secure when someone else is taking care of the critical issues in your life?
- Do you feel you have to ask or coax or cajole others to get what you want?
- Do you understand how the organization's decisions are made?
- Do you feel that you are the only one capable of making the major decisions for your group?
- Do you fear physical, verbal, or emotional confrontation in any of your relationships?
- Do you believe someone else is to blame for your lot in life and that you are a victim?
- Do you feel you have a characteristic that draws discrimination from others?

Style 2: Paternal Manager—The Relational Stage

Manager is moving from a parental style fostering dependency and compliance toward self-confidence with basic relational skill development.

Leadership Style

- Listens to subordinates but reserves decision making for self
- Demands loyalty to superiors
- Insures careful following of the rules

Follower Behaviors

- Feels cared for and protected
- Dependent behaviors
- Views leader as approachable but recognizes that s/he has the last word

Characteristics of this Stage

Starting Point	Well Developed
Beginning competency	Expanding skills
Stranger to the organization	Knows the culture and politics
Dependent on supervisor/leader	Supported by supervisor/leader
Other-awareness	Enlarging self-awareness

Impact of style on group/organization:

This style is appropriate when the leader is highly skilled and the followers are not, such as when a new program is being rolled out in the organization. Relationships are based on fairness and mutual respect. However, rules and protocols are expected to be followed to assure an ordered environment. This style becomes dysfunctional when excessive rigidity and perfectionism is demanded while followers are seeking more autonomy and individual responsibility.

Checking In: To what extent (on a scale of 1–5)

- Do you watch other people to consciously imitate their behavior, to dress for success, or to decide whom to be seen with?
- Is your leadership role model reflective of one of your parents?
- Is your self-concept dependent on how other people feel about you?
- Do you feel that others need to be constantly told what to do, and their performance closely monitored because they don't know quite what to do when left to their own devices?
- Are your social contacts work-related colleagues?
- Are you aware of the specific skills and knowledge that you are striving to develop in order to progress your career?
- Do you feel that your performance as a leader is reflective of all that you are inside?

Style 3: Bureaucratic Efficiency Manager—The Institutional Stage

Manager is moving from competition and control toward cooperation through basic collaboration/team-building skill development.

Leadership Style

- Manages by objectives with a focus on order, clear policies and goals
- Demands respect and loyalty to the institution, its mission and systems
- Delegates only to those who are skilled and loyal to the institution

Follower Behaviors

- Views the leader as approachable and good listener
- Sees tasks and expected outcomes clearly through leader's articulation
- Accepts the exercise of delegated authority in defined areas

Characteristics of this Stage

Starting Point	Well Developed
Controlling others	Increasing self-control
Self-centered ego	Increasing self-awareness
Realistic and competitive	Clear and cooperative
Skilled and striving	Expert and flowing

Impact of style on group/organization:

This level of leadership is appropriate when the leader is highly skilled in an area of specialty and followers are attempting to increase competency in this area. Skills most essential for success are interpersonal effectiveness and professional mastery. The danger of rigidity and resistance to change fosters a "group think" phenomenon, which limits creativity and adjusts performance to meet unique needs of client. On a personal level, at this stage of leadership development a tension is beginning to form between loyalty to the institution and the desire to spend time with family and oneSelf.

Checking In: To what extent (on a scale of 1–5)

- Do you feel competitive about almost everything you do?
- Do you think that power is finite, that is, there is only so much to go around?
- Do you understand and participate in the political games that people in the organization play?
- Do you usually ask yourself first, "How will this affect me?"
- Are symbols extremely important to you, like salary, titles, material possessions, office placement, or number of supervisees?
- Do you think success will make you a better person?
- Do you believe power means being in control of others?

Style 4: Collaborative Manager/Leader—The Enabling Stage

Manager is moving from a work-driven and group focus toward an organizational leader perspective with basic unit management skill development.

Leadership Style

- Caught between demanding efficiency and human needs of staff
- Trying to balance institutional demands with personal values
- Highly skilled as a listener and clarifier

Follower Behaviors

- Willing to express feelings, needs, and expectations
- Spontaneously shares unique perspective in clinical situations
- Demonstrates need for good interpersonal skills

Characteristics of this Stage

Starting Point	Well Developed
Thinking and Doing	Active Intelligence and Being
Reactive	Responsive
Imitates boss or role model	Authentic personal style
Work with people in projects	Lead people and projects

Impact of style on group/organization:
This is a stage of confusion in the developing leader. They are less certain about their beliefs and feelings. A search for new meaning may move the person away from loyalty to the institution toward increased sensitivity to the needs of the staff and self. Decision making may be difficult due to inner conflict, fostering a time of inaction. If one gets stuck here, there is a danger of slipping back into a more bureaucratic and controlling management style.

Checking In: To what extent (on a scale of 1–5)

- Do you take pride in a solid record of competent work?
- Are you sponsoring and celebrating the good work of others?
- Have you consciously chosen to act with integrity?
- Do you think beyond your current job and peers as part of your base of influence, that is, community, professional leadership, political arena?
- Is it important for you to have a natural and personal style that is yours rather than what the organization expects?
- Do you find that the symbols of success do not flatter or motivate you the way they used to?
- Do you utilize both logic and intuition, depending on the situation?

Style 5: Authentic Leader—The Democratic Stage

Leader is moving from career and success focus toward living one's life purpose through basic system building skills development.

Leadership Style

- Very democratic in leadership style
- Has clear vision about how to make institution more humane
- Able to modify rules according to personal conscience

Follower Behaviors

- Good in small group interactions
- Participates as peer in decision-making with patients and colleagues
- Demonstrates need to develop collaboration skills, including conflict management

Characteristics of this Stage

Starting Point	Well Developed
Self-judging	Self-accepting
Anxious and pushing	Calm and allowing
Notices the obvious	True visionary
Tentative about life	Confident of life purpose

Impact of style on group/organization:

This leadership style is ideal for managing a professional group of knowledge workers. Passing through the last stage, the leader now has a new sense of personal creative energy and clear vision for the work of the organization. Because of the high level of interaction amongst staff, support structures must be established to facilitate sharing of ideas and problems in "real time" to maximize team performance. Great demand for the leader's time.

Checking In: To what extent (on a scale of 1–5)

- Do you enjoy guiding, coaching and leading others?
- Are you comfortable with yourself enough that other people's opinions of you do not affect you?
- Do you have a life purpose that reaches beyond yourself and your organization?
- Do you have a deep inner core of spirituality?
- Is your ego getting smaller and less significant all the time?
- Do you consciously give power away by empowering others?
- Do you often laugh at your own foibles?

Style 6: Servant Leadership—Partner Stage

Leader is moving from focus on organizational goals and activities toward living in connection with the public through community building skill development.

Leadership Style

- Concerned with the quality of interaction in the organization and its impact on society as well as with productivity
- Fosters interdependent governance by peer teams on the basis of agreed upon values
- Encourages group decision making as a normal process along with mutual responsibility and collegiality

Follower Behaviors

- Willing to take on responsibility
- Lives and works at high levels of trust and relationship
- Well developed creativity and courage of authenticity

Characteristics of this Stage

Starting Point	Well Developed
Dualistic thinking	Comfortable with paradox
Holds on to power selectively	Powerless
Visible in service	Quiet and unseen in service
Honest	Ethical

Impact of style on group/organization:

Leaders at this level of development have an acute awareness of the rights of all human beings, not just those in the organization. Now decisions are made collaboratively and authority is always used cooperatively. Most essential for sustainability is the capacity to balance involvement in the development of a just and humane organization with ample time for solitude and reflection.

Checking In: To what extent (on a scale of 1–5)

- Do you operate on an inner set of ethical principles that pervade your life?
- Do you identify and understand the role of various individuals and groups in political groupings?

- Are you skilled in teambuilding and art of negotiation?
- Are you open to the attitudes, experiences, and ideas of others?
- Do you have a life purpose that is your guiding influence?
- Are you able to generate alternative solutions to problems in partnership with others?
- Do you see all of life as a paradox?

Style 7: Prophetic Leader: The Universal Stage

Characteristics of this Stage

This level of leadership is rarely found. Leadership and followership are merged; the concepts becoming meaningless. All activity is interdependent in nature and global in concern. The focus is on restoring balance between the world of material goods and the needs of each human being; to work on issues related to ecology, human rights, and reconciliation of conflict, along with the creative and humane use of technology. These leaders are rarely seen or heard as their activity is outside formal systems and processes.

DISCERNING ESSENCE EXERCISE

A Living Example

Nursing is a paradox; you are both a leader and a follower. Many of us work within an organizational setting so we have a leader to coordinate the efforts of the group. Within that reality, we also have our own patient group to manage for the day. This requires all of the management/leadership functions to be applied to the person and the team needed to meet their care needs. Leadership values studies have identified various styles and stages within the discipline. Practice your perceptive skills by studying the five profiles and identifying which leader is: CNO of Health System, Unit Manager, Health Care Consultant, CNO of 150-bed Hospital, Holistic Nursing Consultant. Things to consider regarding their work and client population include the following: unique aspects of their work, inner and outer world focus as it relates to the group the support, amount of autonomy or teamwork required in the role. Their #1 value is their primary motivator.

FIGURE 10.2

Values Profiles for Nurse Leaders

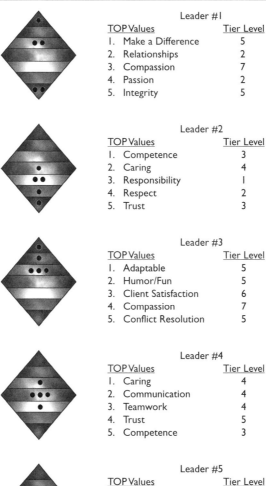

Leader #1

TOP Values	Tier Level
1. Make a Difference	5
2. Relationships	2
3. Compassion	7
4. Passion	2
5. Integrity	5

Leader #2

TOP Values	Tier Level
1. Competence	3
2. Caring	4
3. Responsibility	1
4. Respect	2
5. Trust	3

Leader #3

TOP Values	Tier Level
1. Adaptable	5
2. Humor/Fun	5
3. Client Satisfaction	6
4. Compassion	7
5. Conflict Resolution	5

Leader #4

TOP Values	Tier Level
1. Caring	4
2. Communication	4
3. Teamwork	4
4. Trust	5
5. Competence	3

Leader #5

TOP Values	Tier Level
1. Relationships	2
2. Passion	2
3. Problem Solving	4
4. Caring	4
5. Conflict Resolution	5

Reflective Questions:

1. Are there common values shared between these leaders?
2. What is their style of decision making?

3. How would the top two values of each leader influence their behavior?
4. What nurses would work best for/with each of these leadership styles?
5. Identify your top three Professional Values.
6. What is your leadership style?
7. What behaviors might you develop further to accentuate them even more?

Answers to the Exercise:

The five leaders in Figure 10.2 are:
(A) Holistic Nursing Consultant
(B) Unit Manager
(C) CNO150 bed hospital
(D) CNO Health System
(E) Health Care Consultant.

By focusing on a values cluster profile and sensing into the energy pattern it portrays, you can intuitively perceive the "essence" of the individual, as well as the group they support.

Web Site Resource: This Web site for the Institute for Healthcare Improvement offers examples of projects/programs designed to improve the quality of care in the industry: *http://www.ihi.org*

BIBLIOGRAPHY

Ardaga, A. (2005). *The translucent revolution*. Novato, CA: New World Library.
Armour, J. A., & Ardell, J. (Eds.). (1994). *Neurocardiology*. New York, NY: Oxford University Press.
Armstrong, K. (2001). *Buddha*. San Francisco, CA: HarperCollins.
Berry, T., & Swimme, B. (1992). *The universe story*. San Francisco, CA: Harper Row.
Childre, L. (1999). *The heartmath solution*. San Francisco, CA: HarperSanFracisco.
Ferris, T. (1992). *The minds sky: Human intelligence in a cosmic context*. New York, NY: Bantam Books.
Fisher, B. S. (1996). *The gurdjieff teachings: A compilation a summary*. Prescott, AZ: Subru Press.
Greene, B. (1999). *The elegant universe: Superstrings, hidden dimensions and the quest for the ultimate theory*. New York, NY: Random House.

Guthrie, W. K. C. (1960). *The greek philosophers: From thales to aristotle.* San Francisco, CA: HarperCollins.

Hahn, T. N. (1999). *The heart of Buddha's teaching: Transforming suffering into peace, joy and liberation.* New York, NY: Broadway Books.

Hall, B. P. (1986). *The genesis effect.* New York, NY: Paulist Press.

Harner, M. (1990). *The way of the shaman.* New York, NY: Harper Collins.

Heschel, A. (1956). *God in search of man.* New York, NY: Jewish Publication Society.

Jerison, H. J. (1997). Evolution of prefrontal cortex. In N. A. Krasnegor (Ed.), Development *of the prefrontal cortex: Evolution, neurobiology and behavior* (pp. 118–126). Baltimore, MD: Paul H. Brookes Publishing.

Kaufman, S. (1995). *At home in the Universe.* Oxford, UK: Oxford University Press.

Kuhn, T. (1970). *The structure of the scientific revolution* (2nd ed.). Chicago, IL: University of Chicago Press.

Lao-Tzu. (1992). *Tao te ching: A new english version* (Stephen Mitchell, Trans.). San Francisco, CA: HarperCollins.

Lao-Tzu. (2001). *Tao te ching: The definitive edition* (Jonathan Star, Trans.). New York, NY: Tarcher/Putnam.

Leonardo Da Vinci. (1956). *Leonardo da vinci.* In G. Nichodemi (Ed.), et al. London, UK: Reynal, Williams and Morrow.

Lipton, B. H., & Bertsch, K. G. (1991). Microvessel endothelial cell transdifferentiation: Phenotypic characterization. *Differentiation, 46,* 117–133.

Lloyd, M. C. (1923). *Emergent evolution.* New York, NY: Holt & Company.

MacLean, P. (1993, Spring/Summer). The brain and subjective experience: Question of multilevel role of resonance. *Journal of Mind and Behavior, 18*(2–3), 247–268.

Meyer, M. (1987). *The ancient mysteries: A sourcebook of sacred texts of the mystery religion of the ancient Mediterranean world.* San Francisco, CA: HarperCollins.

Nicholson, R. (1967). *Studies in Islamic mysticism.* Cambridge, MA: Cambridge University Press. (Reprint of 1921 edition: *The Idea of Personality in Sufism,* Cambridge University Press, 1023).

Pannikar, R. (1977). *The Vedic experience: Mantramanjari.* Berkley, CA: University of California Press.

Pearce, J. C. (2004). *The biology of transcendence.* Rochester, VT: Park Street Press.

Plato. (1928). *Symposium.* (A. Niehamas & P. Woodruff. Trans.). Oxford University Press.

Raloff, J. (1998, February). EMF's biological influences: Electromagnetic fields exert effects on and through hormones. *Science News,* 153.

Redfield, J., & Murphy, M. (2002). God and the evolving universe: The next steps in personal evolution. New York, NY: Jeremy P. Tarcher/Putnum.

Rifkin, J. (2009). *The empathic civilization: The race to global consciousness in a world in crisis.* New York, NY: Penguin Group.

Schore, A. N. (1994). *Affect regulation and the origin of the self: The neurobiology of emotional development*. Hillsdale, NJ: Lawrence Erlbaum Associates.

Stebbins, G. I. (1969). *The basis of progressive evolution*. University of North Carolina Press.

Steiner, R. (1969). *Knowledge of the higher worlds and their attainment*. London, UK: Steiner Press.

Stephen, M. (1999). *The gospel according to Jesus: A new translation and guide to his essential teaching for believers and unbelievers*. San Francisco, CA: HarperCollins.

Tarnas, R. (1991). *The passion of the western mind: Understanding the ideas that have shaped our worldview*. San Francisco, CA: Harmony.

Wilber, K. (1996). *A brief history of everything*. Boston, MA: Shambhala.

AFTERWORD

Encouragement for Your Journey

Withdraw into your self and look.
And if you do not find yourself beautiful yet,
do as does the creator of a statue that is to be
made beautiful; he cuts away here, smoothes there,
he makes this line lighter, this other purer, until
he has shown a beautiful face upon his statue.
So do you also; cut away all that is excessive,
straighten all that is crooked, bring to light all
that is shadow, labor to make all glow with beauty,
and do not cease chiseling your statue until
there shall shine out on you the godlike splendour
of virtue, until you shall see the final goodness
surely established in the stainless shrine.
And when you have made this perfect work. . . .
call up all your confidence strike forward
yet a step—you need a guide no longer.

Plotinus

GLOSSARY

Active—an awareness coming from a place beyond the thinking mind

- *Active Intelligence*—moving beyond the concrete thought of logic, analysis, and understanding to an active stance of knowing, which incorporates intuition, intent, and Inner Wisdom
- *Active Observation*—moving from passive looking to an active stance of observation by assessing both the concrete and the subtle body, while entering the nurse–patient experience from the perspective of relationship rather than an interventional viewpoint
- *Active Receptivity*—the Feminine function, an active principle of wholeness, a figure-ground dynamism that exposes the invisible half, giving context and meaning to that which it gently uplifts and holds

Aspects of Nursing—domains, focus, and roles of practice

- *Nursing Science*—realm of concrete thought; the *"evaluator aspect"* of the role focusing on observable and measurable facts, data, logic to guide evidence-based practice
- *Nursing Art*—realm of abstract thought; the *"interpreter aspect"* of the role guided by intuition and active awareness which recognizes pattern and meaning
- *Nursing Essence*—realm of authentic presence; the *"witness aspect"* of the role guided by no thought, which creates a space of active receptivity that potentiates healing

Dinergy—the creative energy of organic growth

Essence of the Divine—the highest manifestation of being a human can express

- *Divine Spark—the core SELF*, a direct extension of the Source, the highest vibrational energy spectrum of humankind
- *Spiritual Ego*—creates the region of the Higher Abstract World at three levels:
  - *Will*—the intent behind the creative impulse, which calls forth a germinal idea and begins to move it toward manifestation
  - *Wisdom*—pure focused attention that links us to intuition, which is the Inner Wisdom of primordial intelligence, the quintessence of all our life experiences

- *Active Intelligence*—the upper sphere of the Thought World, which serves as the gateway into the Higher Abstract World. When contacted through simple awareness, a shift in the focal point from concrete to abstract thought occurs, engaging our intuition and Inner Wisdom
- *Soul—Essence of Being*—home of personal divinity, our unique capacities, and life destiny. It is also home of Inner Wisdom and conscience, which gives direction and meaning to our life

Force-Matter—coalescing energy that is turning into form

Human Energy Fields—the multidimensional human organism

- *Gross Physical Body*—coarsest level, inert mineral machine
- *Vital Etheric Body*—energy wrapper that provides the structural and functional blueprints for the forms and programs of organic structures in the body
- *Desire—Emotional Body*—expresses desires, urges, emotions, and higher aspirations
- *Mental—Reflective Body*—reflects the body of thought, knowledge, and experience
- *Causal Body*—outer sheath of body–mind–spirit that houses the Spirit.

Levels of Reality—our level of consciousness determines reality; increasing awareness creates a more intricate nervous system capable of environmental interaction in a more complex pattern

- *Consensual Reality*—shared perception of things that can be seen or touched, which are validated by the science and culture of the times
- *Inner Reality*—highly individualized perception of inner experiences of fantasies, subjective feelings, emotions, and dreams
- *Core Essence*—a highly developed perception of the subtle energy field behind the form being observed

Prana—Vital Life Force—a form of universal energy, originating from the sun, which is transformed into vitality globules in the spleen to energetically nourish the physical body

Real Power—the ability to create our own reality, to live our own life, and fulfill our destiny. This occurs when we effectively manage both "fast" and "slow" feelings

- *Fast Feelings*—spurred by fear or aggression create swift and decisive movement as they are part of our survival mechanism, housed in the reptilian and mammalian portions of our brain and concrete thought
- *Slow Feelings*—such as stillness and complex memories foster nonaction, are essential for the unfolding of human potential, and are housed in out-of-body consciousness

Seed Atoms—crystal forms of spiritual anatomy, which contain all attributes and knowledge acquired through all evolutions of the consciousness cycles and stored in the Spirit within the Causal Body

- *Seed Atom of Physical Body*—located in left ventricle of the heart, captures holographic pictures of all life events
- *Seed Atom of Vital Body*—located in solar plexus, captures all modifications made to vital blueprints in this lifetime
- *Seed Atom of Desire Body*—located in the liver, records all emotional thoughts and urges as well as higher aspirations
- *Seed Atom of Concrete Mind*—located in frontal sinus, records all thoughts, ideas, and creative ventures within the current life journey
- *Silver Cord*—joins four seed atoms of the personality, connecting all our bodies of consciousness

Shifting the Focal Point—moving the focus of attention from the lower world of concrete thought to the higher world of abstract thought

- *Region of Concrete Thought*—three lower levels of embodied thought manifest in the gross physical body as senses (vital etheric), feelings (desire emotional), and analysis and logic (lower portion of mental reflective)
- *Region of Abstract Thought*—the three higher levels of spiritual consciousness, which include wisdom (focused intuition), intent (will power), and our core SELF (Spirit—our divine spark of life)
- *Mid-Level (fourth) of Thought World*—region of archetypal forces, the place between lower and higher mind where thought crystallizes into form, also the home of the Focal Point whose location is determined by the vibratory level of the person (slower vibration draws focus to concrete thought; faster vibration draws focus to abstract thought)
- *Mind-Body*—an organized cloud of force matter serving as the bridge between the Regions of Concrete and Abstract thought
  - *Concrete Thought*—the lower vibrational sector that serves as our vehicle for thinking, the "i" of thought, emotion, personality, and ego
  - *Abstract Thought*—the higher vibrational sector that serves as the seat of the intuitive mind and "I" of the higher intellect, the spiritual ego and portal for creative, germinal ideas that flow from the field of infinite possibility
  - *Home of the Soul*—our individuality and conscience found in the sixth dimension over the heart chakra
  - *Intuition*—the Inner Wisdom located in the soul that increasingly contributes aspects of our unique potential and provides guidance for us to move down the true path of our identity and destiny

Spheres of Consciousness—human energy physiology includes consciousness at various stages of expression in each human being

- *Objective Universe—Essence of Body*—the concrete world of form; body, personality, and ego
- *Subjective Universe—Essence of Divine*—the abstract spiritual world of being; spiritual ego and core SELF
- *Intermediate Sphere—Essence of Mind*—the intermediate mental world of thought; functions as the Focal Point between concrete and abstract mind
- *Causal Body—Vehicle of Consciousness*—the outer sheath covering body–mind–spirit; repository of essence of all previous lifetimes, home of Spiritual Ego

Spirit of Universal Consciousness—the Universal Spirit is the deepest and most inclusive ground of being. Spirit is the source of all that exists. Spirit is the infinite, creative energy that gives birth to the universe. Spirit is the common source of the world's faith traditions. Spirit is the love that creates and sustains life. The Spark of Life is the Spirit manifest in each person

Vision—the act of seeing

- *Passive Mechanism*—ordinary sight or physical vision using organs of sight
- *Active Mechanism*—perceptive mental vision using a radar-like system

Vitality Globules—etheric corpuscles that provide energy nourishment for the body through force openings (chakras) located in Vital Etheric Body

INDEX

Abram, D., 261
Absolute consciousness, 58–59, 63
Acceptance, 126, 176
Active intelligence, 15, 60, 104,
    108–114, 165–166, 184
Active mechanism, of seeing, 106,
    107–108
Active observation, 53, 104, 105–108
Active receptivity, 5, 104, 114–124
    essence and, 10, 11, 115
All-That-Is, 5, 74, 98, 114, 117, 279
    harmony with, 93, 269
    science discovering, 12
Allopathic medical practices, 65
Ambiguity, 270–271
American Association of Critical Care
    Nurses, values profile of, 189
American Home Health Association,
    values profile of, 189
Archetype, 82
    feminine, 7
Aristotle, 206, 281
Art
    clinical reasoning as, 14–15
    perspective and, 256–261
    physics/science and, 255, 260
    triad dimension of nursing, 10, 14–15
Art of living, 268–269
Assagioli, R., 150
"The aura". See Vital body
Authentic healing presence, 15–18,
    99–100
Authentic leader, 297–298
Authenticity, 96, 148–152, 177–181,
    207, 218–219
Autocratic dictator manager, 293–294

Axial Age, 279, 281
Ayurveda, 69, 137

Bailey, A. A., 162
Balance
    dynamic, 84–87
    personal and professional,
        186–191
Balanced living, and path of
    becoming, 175–205
Balanced wholeness, 168–169
Being, 62
    doing and, 176
    spiritual dimension of nursing,
        95–100
Beliefs, 208
    and control biology, 50
    healing process and, 138
    health, 131–135
    reality shaped by, 254
Bendit, L. J., 139
Bioenergetic system, of human body,
    48, 49–56
Biology
    beliefs and, 51
    cellular development in, 287
    epigenetics, 244
    transcendence, 284–292
Body
    causal, 62, 73–74
    center openings of (chakras), 68,
        80–81
    conceptualization of, 241
    desire/emotional, 69, 70–71, 136
    energy fields of, 47–56
    essence of, 60